613.25
WAL

2|10

Walton, Noah,
  1980-

Ultra-fat to ultra-
  fit.

©2009

| DATE | | | |
|---|---|---|---|
| | | | |
| | | | |
| | | | |
| | | | |
| | | | |
| | | | |
| | | | |
| | | | |
| | | | |
| | | | |
| | | | |
| | | | |
| | | | |

8 |0- 9

# ULTRA-FAT
## *to*
# ULTRA-*FIT*

A Scientist's Rational Approach
to Extreme Weight Loss
and Optimal Fitness

NOAH WALTON, PhD

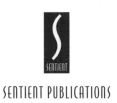

SENTIENT PUBLICATIONS

First Sentient Publications edition 2009
Copyright © 2009 by Noah Walton, PhD

A paperback original

Cover design by Kim Johansen, Black Dog Design
Book design by Timm Bryson

Library of Congress Cataloging-in-Publication Data

Walton, Noah, 1980-
  Ultra-fat to ultra-fit : a scientist's rational approach to extreme weight loss
and optimal fitness / Noah Walton.
     p. cm.
  ISBN 978-1-59181-090-2
  1. Reducing diets—Anecdotes. 2. Weight loss—Anecdotes. 3.
Exercise—Anecdotes. 4. Walton, Noah, 1980—Anecdotes. I. Title.
  RM222.2.W2647 2009
  613.2′5—dc22
                           2009015004

Printed in the United States of America

10 9 8 7 6 5 4 3 2 1

SENTIENT PUBLICATIONS
A Limited Liability Company
1113 Spruce Street
Boulder, CO 80302
www.sentientpublications.com

# CONTENTS

## Musings on Weight Loss

# NOTE

Though all of the individuals mentioned in this book are real, the names and identities of several people have been changed to protect their identity. In addition, "Helen" is a composite of two individuals. Some dates and minor details of events may be slightly inaccurate, victim to the ravages of time and my hazy perceptions in the heat of the moment. Also, it was necessary to reconstruct several conversations from memory, and I have attempted to do so as faithfully as possible.

# ACKNOWLEDGEMENTS

Writing a book is a lot like being the front man for a rock band. You may be the only one everyone in the crowd sees, but you're gonna sound pretty bad without the rest of the group. Here's who's backing me up: Rachel Kamins, my divine editor, who's polished my writing to within an inch of its life. My team of eagle-eyed readers: Croydon Fernandes, Jennifer Hathaway, Susan Heatter and Pavlo Kuzyk, who had the courage to wade through the dreaded rough drafts. Thanks also go to Anne Devlin, Connie Shaw, and all the folks at Sentient Publications who took a chance on a new voice. Last but not least, Mom and Dad, who supported me long after I should have become self-sufficient.

# PREFACE

*A moment's insight is sometimes*
*worth a life's experience.*
—OLIVER WENDELL HOLMES

On a warm day in March, I was sitting at a picnic table on the research campus of Duke University. The pleasant weather had coaxed
me outside, where I was having lunch with a group of co-workers and
friends. One of the latter, a veterinarian named Helen, was recounting
various tales from her days in private practice. At the moment, Helen
was railing against pet owners who let their animals get fat over the
winter.

"It's amazing," she said. "These people come in, their animal looks
like a sausage link, and then they act surprised when I tell them they're
going to have to put Rover on a diet!"

"Wait," I interjected. "You actually put animals on a diet?"

"Sure. Easiest thing in the world. You just don't feed them as much."
This was delivered with the tone an adult takes when delivering a basic
truth to a gullible six-year-old.

"Hold on a second," I said, mad at being chided. "People are animals too, and I know people who have dieted and either didn't lose any
weight or lost it for a while and then gained it back. How can cats and
dogs—also animals, I believe—lose weight 100 percent of the time?"

The table got quieter. Obesity wasn't a taboo subject with this group; most of us were researchers in a lab that studied the effects of obesity in the brain. What was clamming everyone up was the fact that the conversation was straying into a realm that might be a little too close to home for me. I was by far the heaviest person there, well beyond the range of weight covered by lighthearted descriptions such as "chubby," and everyone was afraid that they would inadvertently say something that would hurt my feelings.

Helen, however, was still prepared to play ball. "I've never seen a dog that didn't lose weight on a diet. Dogs *can* do it. People *can* do it, too. They just *don't*."

Although I'd never really tried it myself, I found it difficult to believe that people capable of losing weight didn't just do it. There seemed to be tons of experts and diet plans out there. Surely success in dieting was the norm, and failure the exception. After lunch, I went back to my lab and did a web search on the efficacy of diets. I discovered a recent article[1] suggesting that only one in twenty people was successful in losing and keeping weight off for a period of two years. This was the general consensus among the published studies I could find. Somehow this seemed wrong to me. One in twenty meant that only 5 percent of the dieting population was actually getting it done; you'd almost have better odds playing the lottery.

The next day at lunch, I revealed my findings to the group, and asked Helen to elaborate on why she thought that animals had an easier time dieting than people.

"It's not that they do have an easier time, necessarily. Dogs and cats would be as fat as we all are if they could. They get skinny for only one reason: they don't know how to open the fridge. Think about it—we've all got years of evolution hard-wired into our genes. One of the things we're designed to do is conserve energy in times of surplus. You pack it away when times are good so it's there when they aren't. Now that we've invented grocery stores, there aren't any times of scarcity, so we bulk up. It's natural for people to be fat."

"I think you're forgetting one thing," I replied. "We can open the fridge, but we also have tools at our disposal no other animal has, like willpower and reason." Again, eyes were cast down around the table. No one wanted to suggest that I myself could use a little more willpower and a little less pizza.

Helen shrugged. "You've got biology on one side, and reason on the other. You said one in twenty diets succeeds? I think you have your answer as to which is the bigger kid on the block."

At lunch on the third day, my life changed forever. Everyone was tired of talking about food, evolution, and genetics, but I persisted.

"I don't think who we are prevents us from controlling our actions," I told the group. "I think we're responsible for what we do, because we *are* in control of our lives. I think the reason nineteen out of twenty people fail to lose weight is either because they don't really want it badly enough, or because they go about it wrong. It's not because they can't; it's because they won't."

"Have *you* ever tried to go on a diet?" Helen asked. "It's pretty hard." There was a sharp intake of breath at the table. There it was, out in the open. Fifteen years of fat-person common sense screamed at me to steer the conversation elsewhere, before I embarrassed myself. For some reason, on this day I wasn't quite ready to back down from Helen's implied challenge.

"I'm sure it's tough, but I think I can get myself to do just about anything. Hell, losing weight mostly seems to be about not doing things, like ramming a fork into your mouth," I answered.

"Well," Helen said in a tone that bordered on exasperated, "since you've apparently solved a problem that's vexed modern society for fifty years, why stop there? You can just will your butt into shape and start doing marathons or something. Or ... oh, what are those triple sport things on TV every year?"

"Ironmans?" one of our tablemates suggested, referring to the long-distance triathlons comprising a 2.4-mile swim, a 112-mile bike ride, and a 26.2-mile marathon.

"Yeah, Ironmans," said Helen. "You could start doing them. Be on TV. You'd just will yourself to do it. Simple as that."

The gauntlet had been thrown down, and I have a proud tradition of allowing myself to be easily baited.

"Challenge accepted," I said, not sure if I was bluffing or not. We shook hands and got back to lunch.

Later that afternoon, I got to thinking about our discussion. The exchange had mostly been in jest, and I could easily get out of the agreement by treating it as a joke. But in fact, I wasn't sure I wanted to. Losing weight and getting into shape was an intriguing possibility, the sort of thing I'd dabbled with in my fantasies but never considered seriously. Nor was I terribly enamored of being fat; in the past several years, I had become increasingly unhappy with the state of my life, and I'd begun to suspect that this malaise was directly connected to my ever-increasing waistline. A seed of hope had been planted. *What if I actually did this? Would it be hard? Was it possible? What would it take, and what would it be like?*

I spent the next five years finding out.

SECTION ONE

# TRIAL
# &
# ERROR

# 341

*In order to be effective, truth must penetrate like an arrow—and that is likely to hurt.*

—WEI WU WEI

On March 1 of 2002, I did something I hadn't done in more years than I cared to count: I got on a scale. After flashing double zeroes for three interminable seconds, it announced that I weighed 340 pounds. In truth, the scale read 341 pounds, but I figured my clothes were responsible for some of that.

I felt as though I had swallowed a large, cold stone that had lodged in my stomach. The tiny red numbers hung there, immutable, arousing in me a cold dread, a mixed sensation of panic, terror, and the helplessness a child feels when he's just been busted by an authority figure. There was no chance of a mistake, no hope of rationalizing or negotiating with the number peeking up from between my toes. I was enormous.

Still, to say that this was shocking would be an overstatement. I hadn't joined the ranks of the obese overnight. In fact, I was a typical healthy kid in my early years. I played sports, often staying out until dinner, and generally reveled in the state of perpetual hyperactivity that youth allows. But my idyllic lifestyle began to change as I entered third grade. The marginal hiring practices of North Carolina's public school system dealt me an instructor whose English was flavored by an accent so strong that my uninitiated ears were unable to translate her utterances into useful instruction. I began to struggle with my schoolwork. Fearing for their only child's educational future, my parents registered me at the local Catholic school. This transfer would prove to have a significant and long-lasting impact on my life. Introverted by nature, I was slow to make friends under the best of circumstances, and a mid-year transfer is a social death sentence to a painfully shy child. Left to my own devices, I turned to more solitary cerebral pursuits. Recess, formerly an opportunity for an hour of legitimate aerobic exercise, became a time for reading a book on a swing. My weight began to creep upward.

I did eventually find new playmates. Fate, however, tirelessly conspired to keep me inactive. Coming of age in the late 1980s, my generation was the first to experience home computing. For a ten-year-old, this advancement manifested itself in the form of Nintendo. I spent countless hours perfecting my gaming technique, often with a bag of chips at the ready for pauses in the (in)action. This was excellent exercise for my thumbs but did precious little for my heart and lungs.

Elementary school ended, and middle school arrived. Since school sports eligibility was a year away, I joined the band, and found out I wasn't too bad. Playing the trumpet took priority over everything but girls, and it seemed a prudent decision to abandon team sports to pursue these dual passions full time.

By the time I hit high school, I was one of the better trumpet players in the state of North Carolina. I was also on the wrong side of 250 pounds. I was now more than merely "chubby" or "husky," and for the first time, I began to feel the social stigma attached to oversized individuals. Rather than taking this as a cue to lose weight, I did what came naturally to combat social disadvantage: I made my personality as effervescent as possible. I assumed the role of *de facto* class clown. Serious teachers gritted their teeth each time I opened my mouth, but classmates considered me good for a laugh. As a result of my antics, I was popular enough in high school to have a girlfriend most of the time and enough pals to pass four potentially miserable years in relative comfort.

High schools are small ponds, and I was a strong enough student to be one of the people who would go somewhere. This perception bought me a measure of respect that made my bulbous figure, if not acceptable, at least not a point of derision. Protected from the mockery of my peers, I bided my time, waiting for bigger and better things while only becoming bigger myself.

I managed to deliver on my potential. The combination of low classroom standards in North Carolina and my unexpected aptitude for standardized tests colluded to produce a letter of acceptance from Duke University. Riding high on a sense that I had actually accomplished something, I was more than content to ignore my steadily tightening wardrobe. During my last semester of high school, I took a partial load of classes, and began to make a habit of leaving early to have lunch at an all-you-can-eat pizza buffet.

My weight gain had been so gradual that it had snuck up on everyone, myself included. Friends and family who saw me pack on ten or fifteen pounds a year had failed to say much of anything, out of a combination of the Southern respect for privacy and social tact. My parents had made some mention of it, but I was over-sensitive to criticism and parried their words with sharp rebukes. The only reversal to my weight gain came and went early, the result of a well-intentioned attempt by my father to head off the alarming inflation of his only son. My father offered to take me to see the R-rated movie *Rambo III* in exchange for losing ten pounds. This was a work I (as a ten-year-old) regarded as the peak of cinematic brilliance. Driven by this singular motivation, I wrestled my weight under control and temporarily lost the ten pounds. While I did eventually get to see John Rambo defeat the Russians, the rewards of dieting for health remained lost on me, and my parents' subsequent attempts at pounds-for-prizes deals were met with indifference.

By the time I finished high school, I was the biggest I had ever been. I had grown to six feet, five inches tall, and my height disguised the weight I had added to a point. It was around this time that stress began to creep into my life, contributing further to my weight woes. The summer before college, I took a job as a telemarketer. For eight hours a day, my job was to sell low-quality mail meters to strangers who seemed to share a penchant for verbally abusing me. I fell into the habit of drowning my sorrows in North Carolina barbeque, all the while looking forward to starting a new phase of my education surrounded by people less judgmental than those I spoke to on the phone.

Arriving at college, I was confident that I would be surrounded by mature, driven people, but no one had mentioned that everyone would be so damn fit. I recall moving into the dorms as a freshman and being especially conscious of how great everyone looked. I, on the other hand, was sweaty, jiggling, and out of breath from climbing up three flights of stairs. I found that my old strategy of winning people over with intellect and Aristotelian wit was rather difficult to execute in a dorm that lacked air conditioning.

Starting in a new place, I was dependent on others' meeting me halfway to form new acquaintances. It was truly a surprise when few people bothered to reciprocate my friendliness, despite my best and most creative efforts to engage them. In a heartbeat, I was right back to where I had been in third grade: a shy kid who hung out in his room rather than going to fraternity socials and rallies for civil liberties in countries no one attending had ever visited. The wonderful girlfriend I had in high school was hours away at her own university. I was fat. I was lonely. And I continued to gain weight.

The consequences of being simultaneously surrounded by people and completely socially isolated were far-reaching and severe. Later, I discovered that lab rats placed in social isolation are more susceptible to sickness, suffer memory impairment, and have completely different brain chemistry than their social counterparts. Naively, I thought that

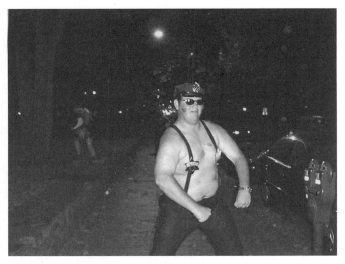

**Halloween, 2000: Coping by making fun of my weight.**

my social isolation would not affect my ability to do well academically. In practice, however, I could not separate business from displeasure. There's a reason every college and university, no matter how small, has a mental health clinic; college is far harder to navigate than a 9-to-5 job when it's difficult to work up the enthusiasm to get out of bed in the morning. The time requirements of a top university are demanding. Perpetually tired and lethargic, I had difficulty getting interested in any of my course material. As a result, my academic performance was uncharacteristically poor. The really scary part was that I just didn't care. The strongest incentive for studying was an aversion to explaining why I did so poorly to the people paying for my education. In the second semester of my freshman year, my neighbor, who was having an even rougher time, had become severely depressed and was failing all of his classes. In order to escape a sheet of Fs, he devised a plan to fake a suicide attempt right before finals. After a standoff with campus police and a few days in the hospital, he succeeded in achieving his goal. I wished I had thought of that trick first.

In hindsight, it's surprising that I finished college without quitting. To almost any realistic person, it would have become increasingly clear after a couple of semesters that things weren't working out, and that it was time to pack it in and do something else. Not I: day after day, week after week, I kept going. To feel better, I ate, became even larger and felt worse. It was a vicious cycle. My perseverance derived not from some noble sense of purpose, but rather from a dumb, intractable stubbornness and a talent for survival. My parent's horror at what I was becoming grew rapidly now; it was especially hard on my father (who, in his heyday, was part of the initial 1970s running boom and remained a pretty fast marathoner). Countless times, he would try to get me to run with him, to come out and exercise, do yard work—anything he could think of to get me to be a little less sedentary. This was to no avail. Ironically, it was my resistance to changing the status quo that ultimately kept me going. I had an idealized notion that quitting was not an option. I was going to finish school without dropping out, transferring, or delaying the experience in any way. As I saw it, this was the way things were supposed to be, and I was going to live the dream whether I wanted to or not.

Laboratory animals often develop coping strategies to minimize or manage the stress of less-than-ideal situations. As did the rodents, so too did I. There were only two lifelines that kept me tethered to the realm of sanity. The first was my girlfriend. I had continued dating my high school sweetheart (in truth, I clung to her like a drowning man to flotsam), and we maintained a long-distance relationship until she moved to the University of North Carolina at Chapel Hill, only eight miles away. Her role in my life was the emotional equivalent of a toxic waste removal engineer, as she remained a constant source of positivity for me even while being subjected to the inordinate amounts of frustration and anger that regularly spilled from my lips. My second source of happiness was my lone hobby—golf. I found playing golf peaceful and liked even more the fact that it allowed me to say I played a sport. Golf probably kept me from turning to alcohol or drugs during this rough time in my life; I spent many a Friday night with my golf clubs at the local driving range. I became a little obsessed, in fact. I was bad, but I didn't care. I signed up for golf in seven of the eight semesters that I was in school. It remains, to this day, the only PE class I've ever voluntarily entered. After my "real" classes were over, I would wander over to the university golf course to chip and putt by myself for hours on end. During my sophomore year, my father moved to Pinehurst, North Carolina, and joined the famous Pinehurst Golf Club. With six different courses at my disposal, I went home almost every weekend to play, returning reluctantly to campus each Monday.

The world rarely takes the day off just because you're having a bad one. I was aware enough to realize that, while I might not care how I did in school *now*, I might at some point in the future. I did the best I could to hold things together. In fact, I was so occupied dealing with my immediate problems that I never considered trying to address what might be causing them. The easiest and most convenient thing to believe was that I just didn't like college. I was fixated on escaping and trading the ivory towers of academia for the steel-and-glass towers of the real world. I decided to graduate in three years instead of four. Ostensibly, this was to save time and money, but in reality, I'm not sure I would have lasted another year.

In the end, I made it through to graduation. Barely. Despite being mired in indifference, I'd adapted to the grade game of college well enough to generate remarkably good results from very little effort, and in my last few semesters I managed to repair the earlier damage to my college GPA. As graduation neared, a single thought pierced the pall that surrounded me: *What now?* I had spent so much time focusing on getting through the present that I had no idea of where I was going or what I was going to do with the rest of my life. I had originally entered college as a pre-med student (despite some veiled warnings about the profession from my parents, both clinicians), but dropped that after (*a*) realizing that I lacked the vigor to earn the high marks medical schools tend to appreciate and (*b*) working in a hospital during my freshman year just long enough to discover that I had an aversion to being around sick people. I'd bounced around aimlessly until I landed in a job as a student researcher in a lab, studying the role of diets high in fat and sugar as risk factors for developing Alzheimer's disease, the irony of which was completely lost on me at the time. I found that I liked the work and the lifestyle of a bench researcher, and could work up little enthusiasm for pursuing other occupations. Essentially by default, I decided to pursue a career in biomedical research.

My first postgraduate job was fairly straightforward. With a minimum of groveling, I convinced the professor I worked for to promote me to a full-time research technician. After years of trying, I had finally reversed the flow of money between myself and Duke University. *Things should be a lot better now,* I thought on my first day of work. I had no homework, a lot of free time, and a good job that supplied me (as a single man) with a comfortable amount of money. And yet, a month after starting the new job, my work performance was stagnating and I felt not one iota better than I did as a student. Nothing was obviously wrong, but I was still clearly bothered by something in my life. So much for my theory that things would improve after college.

Personal malaise yearns to be shared. I began to regularly vent my ill disposition onto friends and family members. By lashing out periodically, I drove away all but my hardiest companions, casting myself into increasingly deeper levels of social isolation and further darkening my own mood. Things came to a head one day when I convinced my girlfriend to accompany me to a golf tournament several hours away from home. During the course of the day, I had one of my frequent mood swings and picked a fight with her. A raging argument ensued, ending when I stormed away, effectively stranding her far from home. Fortu-

nately, I soon returned to my
senses and went back to get her
and smooth things over. This
didn't change the fact that I was
now apparently willing to abandon one of the few people who
could stand me. I realized that I
was socially malfunctioning on a
basic level, and for the first time
in my life, I was obligated to seriously consider whether I was
becoming a bad person.

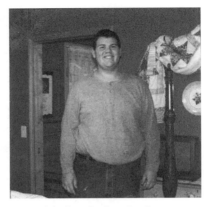

**A month before the diet. Just huge.**

A few weeks after this incident, the fateful series of lunchtime conversations on weight and dieting took place, and my interest and optimism were piqued. Though officially a scientific endeavor, my interest
in losing weight was not purely academic. It was also personal.

It was going to be a hard task. Like a lot of people, I had ignored my
weight problem until it reached epic proportions. A normal body mass
index is 20 to 25. Mine was 40.4, in the range that the medical community refers to as "super obese" and the insurance industry more bleakly
calls "morbidly obese." I needed to go on a diet. I needed to exercise. I
needed to change my lifestyle. I had no idea how to do any of this.

Three hundred and forty-one pounds is a lot of ugly truth. If I focused on the problem, that number represented absolute rock bottom.
On the other hand, when I thought in terms of the solution, that tiny
first step onto the scale had the potential to be my first stride toward a
dramatic transformation of my mind and body.

# Lost in Transition

*See first that the design is wise and just;
that ascertained, pursue it resolutely.*

—WILLIAM SHAKESPEARE

Learning that you're essentially carrying around an entire person in extra fat isn't going to bring a smile to anyone's lips. My first measured thoughts on the matter were something along the lines of *Holy shit! I'm a huuuge bitch!* So-called sensible diet and exercise plans promised a loss of one to three pounds a week. Losing two pounds every seven days, I would reach a normal weight in about sixteen months. When viewed that way, the magnitude of the undertaking became painfully apparent. Walking back into the kitchen for a sandwich and pretending the whole thing never happened looked pretty good. Sometimes I wonder where I'd be if I had done that. Usually, I'm thankful I didn't.

I was a scientist, if an inexperienced one, and I decided to act like it in my approach to losing weight. I decided to treat my extreme weight like a problem I would see in the lab. I started by breaking down the problem into constituent components. I could clearly identify a cause (my weight), an effect (the way it made me feel and function), and a presumptive solution (losing weight). Problem defined, the next step to tackling any problem is to develop a plan to solve it. I needed to map out a strategy in advance, largely because I realized I couldn't trust myself to make solid day-to-day decisions in my current state. Clearly, my thought processes were untrustworthy. People don't get as fat as I was without developing a serious blind spot. Something had made my self-perceptions with regard to weight and health "slippery." Without a firm notion of what I was going to do, I could easily see myself setting out on a diet tomorrow, skipping a few meals, and eventually abandoning the whole endeavor for a capricious reason. But planning a diet is difficult when you have no experience losing weight. Never was it more evident to me than now that I was lacking in both the knowledge and the discipline required to return to the realm of general fitness. I quickly discovered that I was hardly alone in this regard. In America, an estimated $30 to $50 billion is spent annually on weight-loss products by people in the same boat as me.[2]

The wealth of information I found on the subject of dieting was confusing and often contradictory (this was during the heyday of the high-protein, high-fat Atkins diet fad). Over time, I was able to reduce all of the (legitimate) diet advice in the world into one simple, immutable guideline: I needed to take in fewer calories than I burned. Even with that simplification, there was no shortage of ways to go about the task, ranging from highly advertised programs run by the likes of Jenny Craig and Weight Watchers to eclectic (and often dubious) weight-loss systems, each espoused by a single, odd-sounding website. There was an excess of options out there, and I was drowning in them, a classic case of paralysis by analysis.

Lurking behind all of these promises was the basic conundrum that dieticians have been aware of since the 1950s: success in losing weight is the exception rather than the rule.[3] I fancied myself capable of producing an elegant solution (or at least an explanation) for this long-standing problem, one that might be helpful to the larger community. The particulars of my weight problem were common enough, and my findings (and potential solutions) might be broadly applicable. As I would for any other experiment, I followed the venerable hypothetico-deductive model that researchers refer to as the "scientific method." This model has four phases, each of which is applied in turn to the main problem to help identify possible solutions:

1. Gather data and characterize the problem.
2. Hypothesize (or predict) the reason(s) for the problem. This often entails having a solution or desired result in mind.
3. Based on the hypothesis generated, make a prediction, in the form of an "If… then…" statement.
4. Test the prediction with a controlled experiment and analyze the results, observing whether they support or disprove the hypothesis.

Step 1, characterizing the problem, was relatively straightforward. Most people are getting bigger and bigger, unwilling or unable to lose weight, despite efforts to do so. There were a lot of data to back up both of these points: a 2006 report by the Centers for Disease Control found that the prevalence of overweight or obese persons increased by roughly 50 percent between 1960 and 2004.[4] Accordingly, while there are relatively few long-term studies that track people on diets, those that do so agree that regaining weight is the most common outcome. Nor is this regaining of weight gradual: one such study from 1994 found that 87 percent of dieters regain the majority of weight lost within four years of dieting.[5]

An implicit assumption in my weight-loss plan was that being fat is inherently unhealthy, a claim disputed by a small subset of researchers and advocacy groups. In evaluating this issue, I looked into the connection between obesity and health. In fact, an increasingly mainstream movement is aimed at separating obesity from the concept of an unhealthy lifestyle. This idea was relatively new in 2002, but it has gained currency in recent years. For example, a recent study found that fitness was a better predictor of mortality than body fat percentage.[6]

Since my experiment relied on the assumption that thin equaled fit, the question of whether this was indeed the case was critical. In a strict sense, my plan would be to lose weight first, then become fit (in the sense of becoming more athletically competent). I justified my impending actions with two reasons. First, even by alternative measures of fitness, there was no way I could be considered healthy. I sweated when I walked, climbing stairs was hard, and I felt unwell more often than not. Second, opposing weight loss seemed akin to denying global climate change: even if global warming/the link between weight and health is a myth, what do we have to lose by reducing pollution/slimming down? There seemed little to lose, and my mind was made up. In the end, I proceeded with the assumption that fitness and weight were joined at the hip.

On to phase two: formulating my hypothesis for successfully losing weight. At the core of my experimental efforts was a desire to test (and disprove) the idea that people are slaves to their biological yearning to eat, or to bad genetics, for that matter. I hypothesized that, since humans have the faculty of reason, they should be capable of overcoming any vestigial urgings that would oppose weight loss. Already, I could think of two points that supported my hypothesis, at least anecdotally. First, anyone who believed that weight loss was impossible (for any reason) was adopting a defeatist viewpoint, making it unlikely that they would give their absolute best effort and thus creating a self-fulfilling prophecy. Second, although it was a rare outcome, there was the odd person who managed to lose weight and kept it off. Though this didn't prove anything per se, it did suggest that at least a subset of the obese population could effect change on the strength of their desire to do so. After all, if everyone were fundamentally limited in their ability to lose weight by their inherent makeup, how would you explain the successes?

The next step in the scientific process was to make a prediction to test my hypothesis. If I was a logical person (as I believed I was) and if I wanted to lose weight (which I did), then I should theoretically be able to overcome any entrenched biological predilections by dint of my desire to do so in conjunction with my powers of logic. If this strategy succeeded in bringing me to a normal weight, I should be able to continue to use the same principles to continue on to the other side of the physical spectrum—the highest level of elite athletic achievement I could reach.

Why would someone as fat as I was bother with the goal of becoming an elite athlete? Wasn't that looking too far down the road for my own good? Truth be told, it probably was. Clearly, I would only be able to move to the opposite end of the fitness spectrum after I lost a great deal of weight (if, indeed, I was able to lose it in the first place). However, one key assumption in my experiment was that the mind has the capability to push the body to great feats. In order to fully demonstrate this, it was imperative that I not just settle for a merely good outcome, but truly take my physical transformation all the way to the extreme opposite of my current state.

Ideally, my hypotheses and postulations would have been tested in other subjects, through a carefully controlled large-scale clinical study. However, that was unlikely to happen, largely because I had no research grant, nor any prospects for getting one. On the other hand, I was an excellent study candidate myself. I met the prerequisites of being really fat and really motivated to lose weight. I was in an ideal position to record my feelings and events as they happened throughout the experiment so as to provide insight into the process of weight loss and the transition from obesity to a high level of athleticism. Working alone had other benefits. I had little idea what the journey would entail, and it seemed likely that I would be making some things up as I went along. This wasn't good science, but it was unavoidable in discovering what actually worked for weight loss. It seemed wrong to involve others in a process that I didn't yet understand very well. I had a feeling I would be making a lot of mistakes.

As I began to design this grand experiment, I was also in the process of pursuing additional training in science. My job as a research technician had been satisfying enough, but Duke held some bad memories for me, and I felt I would need more stimulating challenges sooner or later. If I was to remain in science, I decided, I should obtain another degree, and so I applied to several PhD programs, eventually accepting a slot beginning that fall at the University of Florida. The thought of more school grew much less daunting as my plan for altering my physique became more concrete. Already, in some small ways, I heard whisperings of my former confidence creeping back. Naturally, the prospect of making a fresh start where I wasn't known as the fat guy was also a powerful motivator.

A secondary goal of my experiment was an exploration of why existing diets were so ineffective. It seemed to me that everyone had a method, regimen, or system for weight loss that promised to make you thin (and happy) if you just followed its rules. Many of these seemed efficacious and sensible. Theoretically, I would have assumed that people would respond well to these systems, as we are raised to follow directions. Yet this was clearly not the case. I wanted to know why there was a high degree of noncompliance and recidivism among dieters. It wasn't that people didn't care about losing weight: at any given moment, between 15 and 35 percent of Americans report being on a diet.[7] In exploring why dieting was so difficult, I hoped to discover how to make people more effective in achieving their weight-loss goals.

The central pillar of my initial strategy would be a diet that put me in a daily calorie deficit, allowing me to burn excess bodyweight to compensate. Not knowing any better (and more than a little afraid to screw things up by being creative), I decided to try the classic balanced diet: plenty of fresh fruits and vegetables, and no sweets, fried food, or alcohol. I would eat smaller, more frequent meals (but never too late at night), count my calories, and exercise. It was the plain vanilla diet you would expect any nutritionist to trot out during an initial consultation.

I had it on good authority from the weight-loss establishment that this would be effective.

In retrospect, it seems likely that, had I actually attempted this method, I would have failed miserably. To the average obese person, the classic diet is like communism: it looks good on paper, but it usually doesn't work when put into practice. The biggest obstacle would be adapting to a 180-degree change in eating habits. The last vegetable medley I had eaten was a fried potato covered with ketchup. I ate huge meals at odd hours, had no concept of portion control, and got 90 percent of my calories from refined sugar and simple carbohydrates. After three days of the classic diet, I would probably have gone into shock from the trauma to my digestive system.

Serendipitously, before I could attempt this doomed plan, help arrived in the form of an unorthodox alternative. On the eve of the first day of my diet, my supervisor walked in, excitedly describing a new study[8] on the effects of various diets on the function of the brain (a topic of particular interest for our lab). In this study, my advisor explained, scientists compared groups of mice that were either fed normally or placed on one of two experimental diets. The first experimental diet was very close to the diet I was planning: each day, the mice were fed about two-thirds of the calories they would need to maintain their bodyweight. With insufficient calories to burn, the mice predictably shed weight. The second experimental diet being tested was a little more radical: the mice were given absolutely nothing to eat (with an unlimited supply of water) for a period of twenty-four hours. On the second day of the diet the (presumably starving) mice were given an unlimited supply of food, and were free to eat as much as they liked for the following twenty-four hour period. On the third day, all food was again removed, and the process was repeated so that animals were allowed to eat only on alternating days. Both diets were maintained for about three months before the outcomes for the control and experimental groups were compared.

I was struck not by the neurobiology but by the weight-loss aspect of the study. Just like a dog placed on a diet by its owner, mice on the first experimental diet lost weight in a predictable manner as a result of constant caloric restriction. These mice were deprived of one-third of their normal caloric intake; each day, an animal on this diet ate about two-thirds, or 67 percent, of what it was used to consuming. On the second experimental diet, animals were first fasted, eating zero percent of what they required during a normal day. The next day, these animals were given access to unlimited amounts of food. After a day of starvation, the hungry mice gorged themselves on the abundance of available food. In fact, they typically ate 180 percent or more of what they would normally consume.

Hmmm…

I did a few quick calculations. If a mouse on the experimental diet eats nothing one day and almost twice what it normally does the next, it's eating more than an animal on a conventional diet over the same two-day period:

Intermittent Fasting Diet:

$$\frac{(0\% + 180\%)}{2 \text{ days}} = 90\% \text{ of normal food intake per day.}$$

Conventional Diet:

$$\frac{(67\% + 67\%)}{2 \text{ days}} = 67\% \text{ of normal food intake per day.}$$

The results were clear: on average, mice placed on an alternate-day-fasting diet actually ate significantly more than animals placed on a conventional diet. Of course, this was nothing to get excited about if the two diets differed in weight-loss results. But they didn't: both groups of mice lost weight!

This study had not been performed on human test subjects, probably because of the difficulty of convincing a group of sane people to fast repeatedly over a long enough period to produce any meaningful weight loss; it would just be too hard for the average person to do. But my interest was piqued. In theory, if I was willing (and able) to fast every other day, I would be able to eat more food and, even better, the same food that I was used to. It seemed too good to be true, yet I had a soon-to-be-published study suggesting otherwise.

Whether alternately eating and fasting was sustainable, or even possible, was a big "if" to deal with. I had never gone without food for more than twelve hours, and that was only for the sake of blood work at the doctor's office. Even then, the unpleasantness of being that hungry was distinct and memorable. Still, the more I pondered things, the more I thought this approach could work for me. It was drastic, flamboyant, and it appealed to my individualistic predisposition not to follow the herd of conventional dieters. In addition, intermittent fasting seemed to offer me two practical advantages over the standard diet I had previously favored. First, the severe nature of intermittent fasting was likely to produce fast results, which would presumably help me stay motivated. And in a similar vein, it seemed likely that alternate-day fasting would be easier to cleanly adhere to than a more conventional diet. My rationale was that fasting required less "active maintenance" (i.e., thinking about calories, portion control, selection of healthy foods, and meal frequency) than a conventional diet. If you're going to mess with something as basic as food consumption, shouldn't you keep the changes you make as uncomplicated as possible? What, exactly, are the advantages of counting points or carbs or measuring portions constantly when you're clinging to your last scrap of discipline?

While I was enthusiastic, I also saw several potential negatives, all reasons why a system like this one would not be offered up to mainstream dieters. For one thing, it probably wasn't sustainable after the target weight was achieved. I'd eventually have to come up with a "phase two" diet, even if phase one worked. But dealing with how to *stay* thin sounded pretty good from where I currently sat. Second, while I didn't think this was physically dangerous, I saw the potential for acute emotional and mental unpleasantness after a day-long fast. Third, I could see this diet crimping my lifestyle. Food plays a key role in social interactions. It's nigh on impossible to take a girl out to dinner and explain why you're sitting there staring at her without eating anything.

In the end, none of these reasons were deal-breakers. There are pros and cons to almost every plan; you can debate them forever, or you can go ahead and try something. I was excited about this particular diet and motivated to get started. My instincts told me to go for it. If it didn't work, I could try another approach, but it seemed imperative to just do something, anything. I boiled down my approach to the following rule, which I wrote out:

1.  Fasting will run on alternating days, from midnight to midnight. On the fasting days, no food will be eaten (including non-caloric substances like mints, gum, or the like). Only water will be consumed. On non-fasting days, any food in any amount may be eaten. The diet will be repeated on this cycle until a healthy weight is reached.

Underneath this dictum, I wrote a number (2) for the next rule, only to realize that there was no need for it. There really wasn't a way to ambiguously define this plan. This total lack of room for interpretation was exactly what I found so appealing about the diet. I was going to come after my problem in a very straightforward, aggressive manner. Frankly, I was more than a little angry at my fat for the problems it had caused me, and I couldn't wait to start putting the hurt on my rolls of blubber. In that spirit, I decided to start the diet immediately, beginning at the stroke of midnight.

I awoke the next morning, raring to begin my new and improved life. Within an hour, I had already blown it. I promptly forgot I wasn't eating and broke my fast at our weekly lab meeting. Having tainted the entire day by this folly, I sat through the meeting in red-faced embarrassment and waited for my "do-over." The next morning, just to be safe, I wrote "No Eat!" on the back of my hand with a Sharpie. This time, and every other day for the next six months, I remembered.

# Life in the Fasting Lane

*Every adversity, every failure, every
heartache carries with it the seed of an
equal or greater benefit.*

—NAPOLEON HILL

Fasting, day one. I woke up feeling OK. As on a standard workday, I drove the eight or so miles from my home in Chapel Hill to Durham, parked illegally at Duke's golf course, and took the bus about a mile across campus to the research building in which I worked. The previous day aside, I wasn't much of a breakfast eater at that point in my life, so I made it until lunchtime without really sensing anything out of the ordinary within my body. I was going along on cruise control and then—BAM! The habitual craving for lunch hit me like a freight train. Discovery number 1: It's amazing how accustomed we are to obeying our body's command to eat. I actually stood up and had my jacket on before I realized that lunch was not on the proverbial menu today. To satisfy my hunger, I decided to drink some water, whereupon I made the unpleasant discovery that water, if anything, made me hungrier.

Discovery number 2: Food plays a huge role in our social lives. Having nothing better to do with the time, I worked through lunch alone, abandoned by co-workers who had left to forage at the nearby cafeteria. The irony of being further socially isolated by my attempt to lose weight was not lost on me. In all fairness, joining my friends was a possibility, but the prospect of sitting at a table watching others eat while fielding their questions about why I wasn't also doing so seemed less than tantalizing.

I've never liked the term "hunger pang." It sounds far too transient and far too civilized, a temporary inconvenience at most. The sensations of hunger I now felt were unrelenting, taking the form of deep, pulsating commands from my stomach to go eat. Immediately. Forthwith. Without delay. These messages were soon supplanted by the more plaintive sounds of my stomach rumbling—softly at first, and then more audibly. During the afternoon, a couple of my co-workers actually heard the noise and asked if everything was OK. I had no idea, I said, which inevitably led to explaining to them what I was doing. The cat was out of the bag and I was now officially on the record. My co-workers looked at me as if I were crazy, possibly dangerous. They were definitely wrong about the "dangerous" part. Discovery number 3: Not eating for a long time makes you feel very, very weak.

Around four o'clock I discovered the first good thing about fasting, when I was able to negotiate an early release because I had worked through lunch. This led to discovery number 4: Increased free time is not something you want when you're trying to forget that you're not eating. After returning home, I went up to my room, determined to simply kill time. Discovery number 5: Trying to distract yourself from hunger is as effective as telling someone with diarrhea to control his bowels. I tried reading, watching TV, and listening to music. Nothing helped. I contemplated going to the movies, but I thought I might pass out in the car and kill myself, on an especially low note. I wound up lying on my bed, watching the clock like a spinster on a Friday night. At one point I resolved to wait until midnight and chow down the second I was allowed to. But eventually, I lapsed into an uneasy sleep, not entirely sure I would make it through the night in my weakened state. As I slumbered, I dreamt I had fallen into a giant tank of nacho cheese and was drowning. I woke up, realized what I had been dreaming about, and tried my damnedest to fall back asleep and reclaim the imagined taste of imitation cheddar.

The next day of the diet was *much* better. I stopped at a bakery on the way to work and gobbled up a couple of bagels. In hospital delivery rooms, mothers are given several pain medications, one of which promotes temporary amnesia. The rationale behind this is to make the mothers forget the pain of childbirth. Cinnamon-sugar bagels became my miracle amnesia drug; once the food hit my system, all was once again right with the world, and by lunchtime the memories of the previous day were faint.

And so a new eating pattern was created. Days when I could eat were generally happy ones. I quickly fell into a routine: lots of carbs in the morning to get me feeling human again, lunch wherever my lab-mates decided to go, and then dinner usually at an all-you-can-eat salad bar near my house (a compromise between my love for large quantities of food and my respect for the "eat your vegetables" commandment drilled into me at a young age). The best part of the diet was that, while it was on occasion very trying, it was free from difficult choices. On any given day, I was eating either nothing or whatever I wanted. In stark contrast to the grinding discipline of a classic diet, the periods when I was able to eat freely emotionally recharged me and kept me going on the hard days.

Naturally, there were a few consequences to what I was doing. The obvious psychological strain was accompanied by some disturbing physical alterations. By the third or fourth day of fasting, amazing things were happening to my body. Unfortunately, few of them were pleasant. Drastic metabolic alterations occur when someone used to more than 6,000 calories a day slashes that number to zero on a regular basis. First and foremost, I was forced to rely on an entirely new source of energy. Human beings typically metabolize relatively simple sugars as immediate fuel sources. Carbohydrates can be quickly converted into constituents for rapid use, while protein and fat (including stored fat, my old nemesis) are converted more slowly, as one might expect of a reserve source of energy. Each day that I fasted, I would run out of carbohydrates to burn by mid-afternoon. I was reduced to running on stores of fat and protein.

This is, of course, the point of pretty much every diet, and some diets (like Atkins) are actually predicated on using fat and protein as primary sources of fuel. Nor was the underlying biochemical process terribly uncomfortable; I wasn't exactly having a sugar crash each afternoon (quite the opposite; I had a lot more energy than I'd thought I would), but my body was breaking down large amounts of fatty acids to keep me running. The sudden, repeated withholding of all sources of nutrition did not buffer the burning of protein and fat with even a small supply of carbohydrates. Practically, this meant I was producing lots of molecules called ketones as waste products. There are only two things the average person needs to know about ketones: they get into your breath, and they stink to high hell. Imagine the worst halitosis you can think of and multiply it by two, and you've got an idea of the toxic fumes I was spewing on a bi-daily basis. Short of breaking down and eating something, there wasn't much I could do. Mints and gum were forbidden by my plan, but they would have done no good anyway, since they wouldn't address (or even mask) the source of the bad breath. Like everything else so far, this was a mixed development. Clearly I would not be meeting many women while on this diet, but you learn who your real friends are when you're having a rough day and have rotten breath to boot.

In another bizarre physical development, my left shoulder blade started to ache mildly, and it would continue to do so intermittently for the next six months. To this day, I have no explanation for why this happened. My best guess is that my body was either punishing me for punishing it, or it was tremendously pleased by the change and was patting me on the back really hard.

I was simultaneously riding an emotional rollercoaster that departed each and every day I did not eat. I would start out normally in the morning, but my emotions would slowly devolve into a neurotic mess as my stomach emptied, my shoulder ache returned, and my breath began to sour. I would fly into tantrums that, after proper nutrition was administered, would seem utterly ridiculous. Why I wasn't fired from my job for gross insubordination remains unclear. Those closest to me knew that my emotional weather now ran on a predictable two-day cycle, which probably made me easier to deal with than before. Previously, I had been angry and moody at random; now I was only that way a regular 50 percent of the time. Progress, indeed. All told, I considered these symptoms perfectly acceptable, given the importance of what I was doing. Especially after I started seeing results.

# Seeing Results

*The distance of the road to success becomes shorter as soon as you take the first step.*

—GREG PHILLIPS

As I continued to diet, I began to appreciate the unique challenges faced by the dieter, which go beyond those faced by people attempting something like quitting a bad habit. In particular, the lengthy time frame required to achieve a weight goal can be particularly daunting, especially when it comes to finding motivation to continue plugging away. But willpower is not so finite as we might think, and it can come from many sources. For me, there was no substitute for simply achieving results. The scale, as I was coming to learn, can be a double-edged sword. It can tell you an unpleasant truth and deflate you by revealing that your hard work is not paying off, or it can give you an almost unimaginable boost of confidence in the efficacy of your chosen tactics. Above all, the scale tells you the truth.

Whatever the emotional impact of the message, the scale is incapable of deception; it has no agenda and acts only as an objective reporter of facts. To a person recognizing his need to diet, the scale will be the first one to deliver the bad news. A crucial first step in dieting is accepting and acknowledging this information as the truth. Indeed, no truer feedback can be found, and the successful dieter makes a habit of validating his methods against the findings of the scale. I needed to learn how to listen to the scale. Fat is incredibly high in energy (a person would have to walk upwards of thirty miles to burn a single pound of fat), and weight loss is a slow process. Day-to-day fluctuations are both expected and explainable. However, results obtained over a period of time give a long-term trend and, thus, an accurate idea of progress. For these reasons, I didn't want to jump on the scale every day, troubling myself over every ounce gained or lost. In fact, I didn't even buy a scale. I checked my weight every weekend when I traveled home. This spacing between weigh-ins proved sufficient to level out the minute daily variations in body weight and give me a sense of the overall trend.

After a week on the diet, I'd lost about five pounds. This was great news and even better motivation. To be honest, there's really not that much difference between a 340-pound man and one who weighs 335. To me, though, two things were gained from this initial weight loss: the results validated my diet as being effective, and I knew that I was making headway. I could now say, for the first time in a long while, that I was slimmer than I had been a week ago. I was still terribly heavy, but I had put a dent in the problem.

From a motivational standpoint, positive feedback in success has been well documented. There is an oft-referenced (albeit sparsely documented) experiment from the 1950s, usually attributed to the venerable Dr. Curt Richter of Johns Hopkins University, in which scientists attempted to quantify the effect of hope. Two groups of rats were placed in buckets of water, forcing them to tread water to stay afloat. One group of rats was briefly "rescued" from the bucket before being returned to the water. These rescued rats treaded water far longer before drowning than their savior-less counterparts. Hope—for future rescue, in this case—is ascribed as the mechanism behind the disparity in effort. For me, the principle was the same. The scale had not only validated my unorthodox approach, it had inspired me to continue into the next week of dieting. I was willing to put up with the highs and lows of my unusual system if it generated results. Going into week two, I thought that if I could put together enough weeks of steady weight loss, I would really be able to chip away at the big problem.

At my second weekly check-in with the scale, I had lost more weight: six pounds this time. The next week I lost another four, and the week after that, five. Losing twenty pounds in under a month officially gave my little diet plan some credibility. Outside of work, I hadn't told a soul; I was waiting for people to notice, while enjoying my secret source of pride. I found myself covertly marveling at how much less weight I now carried. Whenever I found myself in a Home Depot or Lowe's, I would wander out into the gardening section and try to find a twenty-pound bag of mulch or sand to hoist, amazing myself with how heavy it was.

After two months of steady dieting, I was now looking for fifty-pound bags of mulch to lift—I weighed less than 300 pounds for the first time since high school. People finally began to ask me if I was on a diet. The fact that a sixth of my body had disappeared into thin air before people began to notice was a testament to how fat I had been. I was confronted with a wonderful new crisis: my clothes (particularly my pants) had become too large. At my peak, I was pushing a 48-inch waist, and now I was into the low forties. In a show of support, my parents offered to take me shopping for new clothes. During the trip, I told them not to buy me too much, because I was going to need an even smaller size soon. Through a constant, measured effort I was steadily reducing the size of my body, averaging a little less than five pounds of weight loss per week, with no end in sight.

The rush of self-esteem accompanying weight loss must be felt to be truly understood. My willpower was bulletproof; I could fast through dinner in mixed company with only a minimum of temptation. The positive feedback from those around me was also incredible. People are used to seeing themselves in the mirror every day, so the minute changes in our body composition over time often occur too slowly to be appreciated. Only through the comparison of photographs and the comments of those who see you less frequently do you really get a sense of how your appearance has transformed. I set a weight goal for myself: I would continue my diet until I weighed 250 pounds (at the time, this was my best guess at what constituted a healthy weight). I thought if I could just hit that number, I would be healthy once again.

No sooner had I set a tangible weight goal than I hit my first real bump in the road. As I've said, the scale is the best tool for revealing the efficacy of one's approach to weight loss, and my scale had begun to frown on my efforts. One weekend I stepped on the scale and realized that I'd only lost one pound since the last weigh-in. One measly pound. The week before I had lost three, and the week before that, only two. Something was wrong. I was killing myself to lose weight. I was still religiously following my diet—I hadn't cheated once. In fact, I'd actually stepped up my efforts. In the early days of the diet, I would gorge myself when I was allowed to eat freely, partly as a knee-jerk reaction to being very hungry and partly in anticipation of the fact that I was soon to be without food again. As weeks passed, I had taken more ownership in what I was accomplishing, and I found it increasingly difficult to justify deliberate overeating when I'd worked so hard the day before. As a result, my eating habits were starting to change. Now, though, my efforts were running out of steam. Considering that I still weighed about 285 pounds, at the rate my weight was decreasing there was no way I was going to make it to 250.

I was confused by this and felt more than a little cheated. I was doing all of the right things. Why were they suddenly not working? In retrospect, this slowdown heralded the end of the first stage of my experiment, the loss of the easy pounds. This was simple to explain scientifically: I had changed my diet and had burned excess bodyweight as a result. But the body is loath to burn fat unnecessarily and will cling to every last pound and fight for every last ounce. I had unwittingly adapted to my reduced energy intake by slowing my metabolic rate. I had also lost in excess of fifty pounds, which meant that my body required almost a thousand fewer calories per day to operate. These two factors combined produced a dramatic cessation of weight loss.

A plateau in weight can mire the determined dieter in doldrums from which escape proves impossible. Here's why: A stall in weight loss puts pressure on your methods, which puts pressure on you when you're already strained to the breaking point by adapting to this new way of life. Too much stress produces predictable attempts to avoid the stress's source—in this case, the diet. To avoid this pitfall, I needed to do something to get moving again, and fast. To break through to the next level of a healthy lifestyle, it was now time to raise my metabolic rate by adding the next piece of the puzzle: exercise.

Exercise, it should be known, is the bitter arch-nemesis of the rotund. Exercise and I shared a history fraught with mutual disdain and one-sided suffering. High school gym class had embarrassed the last vestiges of athletic inclination out of me, as I failed countless assessments of physical fitness in front of my peers. As an adult, the last real exercise I had gotten was on a summertime trip to the mountains of North Carolina in 2001. My girlfriend had expressed an interest in going caving (essentially, spelunking without the ropes). The brochure made it look easy, and the guides assured me that even a person of my height and weight would have no trouble navigating the confined spaces of the caverns. Liars, all. Since that day, I have run many races, many of them considered insanely extreme by the general public, but rarely have I been as completely exhausted as I was the moment I staggered out of that godforsaken hole in the ground three hours after entering. I could barely manage the quarter-mile walk back to the car. The fact that my girlfriend and I had been partnered with a group of athletic fifteen-year-olds did nothing for my mood, nor did the fact that I had been literally stuck in several tight spots during the ordeal. In a powerfully irrational moment, I had vowed never to exercise again.

Despite these past setbacks, I had begun to toy with the abstract notion of starting to exercise again, much in the way a former jock talks aimlessly of "getting back into things." It wasn't that I had grown fonder of the idea of exercise. Ideally, everyone would be able to easily lose weight without it. But I'd become accustomed to watching the numbers on the scale dwindle each week, and I was now afflicted with a blinding urge to keep them moving down. I would have drunk pond scum if it would help me lose weight. Exercise was an unknown to me. Having been sedentary throughout my entire adult life, I had scant firsthand knowledge of the dramatic effects that regular exercise could exert. Sometimes, though, even when we lack the knowledge to make good decisions, fate cuts us a break and intervenes.

# Running on Fried Chicken

*I believe it's called jogging or yogging.*
*It might be a soft j. I'm not sure, but*
*apparently you just run for an extended*
*period of time. It's supposed to be wild.*

—RON BURGUNDY, *ANCHORMAN: THE*
*LEGEND OF RON BURGUNDY*

The following Monday, I woke up unaware that I was about to undertake the next phase of my journey. The day began unremarkably. I drove the eight miles between Chapel Hill and Durham and parked in my usual spot at the university golf course. I walked to the bus stop and waited for the bus to arrive. It was summer now, and I had a little more than three months to go before moving to Gainesville to begin my doctoral studies at the University of Florida. Over the summer months, Duke hosted a large number of sports development camps for high school students, and my bus stop was near the outdoor complex where they often trained. No more than a stone's throw away, groups of soccer players were scrimmaging. Seeing the kids play summoned fond memories of my younger, more active days. Researching Gainesville, I had found that my soon-to-be home supported a well-developed adult soccer league, and the yearning to play again had become more pronounced as I decreased in weight. Seeing these soccer players drew my priorities into focus: my goals weren't the simple loss of pounds; I wanted to prove that I could push myself to become extremely physically fit. It occurred to me that, in order to achieve this lofty goal, I might actually benefit from exercising sooner rather than later.

There was still no sign of my bus, and I was suddenly restless. The day was cool, and my legs felt springy and unusually powerful, likely because they were carrying much less weight than they were used to. An idea hit me:

*Noah, why don't you run to work? Don't think about it. Just do it. Go.*

I took the first step of my running career that morning at 7:50 a.m. It's easy to remember the exact time, because work started at eight. My building was exactly one mile away, and I assumed that ten minutes would be plenty of time for me to get there.

As it turned out, I was late.

My first effort at running ended about four hundred yards from where it began, because I was going to throw up on myself if I ran one more step. It was amazing how I had gone from feeling so great to feeling so bad so quickly. It was almost as though the sudden activity triggered the physical equivalent of a manic-depressive episode. As I waddled along initially, things had felt so right. I felt the strongest conviction that this was another step in taking back control over my body. Less than five seconds later, my body called in to report that, in fact, all was not well. An uneasy feeling of discomfort spread from my lungs into my sides, and then to my stomach. As if I were wearing a corset pulled too tight, I could no longer take in a full breath, and I was left gasping for oxygen. The feeling intensified until it felt like I was in an all-out sprint, even though I was barely jogging. Physiologically speaking, this wasn't far from the truth. In the previous fifteen years, my body was seldom forced to deal with such strenuous activity, and was unaccustomed to handling the increased workload. My heart and lungs were unable to efficiently deliver oxygenated blood to my equally shocked (and accordingly greedy) muscles. The result was a hypoxic state: I was effectively drowning in broad daylight.

At the time, I had no use for such scientific explanations; I just needed to breathe. I slowed to a walk, but I was determined to cover the
distance on foot one way or another. Seven-year-old kids in gym class
could run a mile. I could at least keep trying. After several minutes, I felt
sufficiently recovered to start running again. Several times, I repeated
the same sequence: I ran until I thought I would collapse, then dropped
back to a walk to regain my strength. If my lungs were autonomous beings, they would have each drawn daggers and cut their way out of my
chest, to move on to a host body that promised never to subject them
to such ridiculous activities. As it was, it only *felt* like they were sawing
their way free from my ribcage. My heart was beating so hard it seemed
to be ricocheting between my ribs and my spine. My progress was
laughable, but I was dogged in my intent to run as much of the distance
as I possibly could and, eventually, I reached my building.

I must have looked horribly comical (or perhaps comically horrible)
finishing my first "run." I was a jiggling, florid wreck with the shambling
waddle of one perpetually lacking in balance. I ground to a halt and
doubled over, fighting off a very credible wave of nausea. I had covered
exactly one mile in fourteen minutes, including four or five minutes of
walking and quite a bit of hyperventilation. I was not dressed for running: I had on khaki shorts and a billowing golf shirt, both of which
were now streaked with sweat from the effort. My shoes were well-worn
tennis flats, providing no support for the pounding I had inflicted on my
knees and ankles. Everything hurt, but I had finished what I started.

Ten minutes later I was in the bathroom, cleaning myself up, still
trying to get my heart rate to retreat to a comfortable level, and con-
templating what had just happened. Specifically, I was wondering why
something so intensely unpleasant was supposed to do me good. But
as of late, I had found that pretty much anything that felt unpleasant
turned out to be good for me. Dieting was a mild but constant pain in
the butt, and it produced results. The longer my diet lasted, the less

unpleasant reducing my caloric intake had become, as my weight decreased in accordance with my reduced food consumption. In effect, I had made a permanent change to my lifestyle and was no longer dieting in the conventional sense. Having made this dietary change, I would now have to do something else to continue to make progress. I hoped that exercise would become more tolerable as I became accustomed to it. For the moment, however, there would be no gain without some pain.

Every day after that first morning, rain or shine, eating or fasting, I would park my car a mile from work, take a deep breath, and set off. In the beginning, I still couldn't run the whole distance continuously, but each day I would run a little farther than the day before. These were ugly, shuffling efforts, but I was improving on almost a daily basis. A week after I started, I was finally able to run the full mile. Even better, my weight had begun to fall again. That sealed it: whether I was ready for it or not, exercise was now a part of my life.

I felt a very abstract sense of satisfaction after each run (usually not during the run itself). Each effort was a tiny microcosm of a lifestyle change, a tiny struggle in and of itself. Each time I stepped out the door to exercise, I wondered whether I would finish what I set out to do or end up compromising my goal for the day. Usually, whether I achieved my goal was up to me—an empowering thought. Whenever I finished something I had started, I felt I had scored a tiny victory. I vowed to continue running every day.

A sad reality about implementing an exercise program while obese is that, when working out, you become *more* subject to the ridicule of others (who are, 99.9 percent of the time, ensconced in a moving vehicle). The illogical timing of those who chose to express their opinion of my size was one of those things that made me shake my head. You have a problem with large folks and can't keep your thoughts to yourself? Fine. But if you hate fat people so much, why the hell would you choose to ridicule one while he exercises? Think that's going to encourage him to keep trying to slim down? I comforted myself by assuming that anyone who yells at overweight exercisers from a car is of subnormal intelligence. And take it from me: there are a lot of stupid people out there.

As summer peaked, I was making headway, but still weighed north of 250 pounds. North Carolina in July is no place to be an overweight novice runner, but I was doing the best I could. I had built myself up to the point where I could run one mile to work and one mile back at the end of the day. When I had conquered that distance, I managed to find an alternate route that stretched the run each way even further. On average I would be honked at, hassled, or heckled once a day, usually by a clever motorist who was unable to suppress his wittiness in response to my free-swinging man breasts or bounding stomach. In the midst of the criticism, I discovered something about myself: I no longer cared what anyone else thought. This was perhaps the first time in my life I could honestly say that was the case.

This is not to say that I was not self-conscious about the appearance of my body. As I lost weight, I would pore over my appearance in the mirror for signs of slimming. The outline of a rib, the earliest vestige of a collarbone, the lessening of a chubby cheek—all were harbingers of my body's emergence from the layers of fat that trapped it. It was as though I were both an archaeologist and my own dig site. I was leaving for Gainesville in less than two months, and if I worked very hard, I would be able to show up reasonably slim.

To that end, I stepped up my efforts yet again, pushing my capabilities on a daily basis. During the workweek, I began combining the short runs to and from work into a single longer run in my neighborhood, partly to take advantage of the cooler night air and partly to avoid the concerned expressions of my co-workers that greeted me each morning when I arrived inexplicably sweating and disheveled. By summer's end, I could run almost four miles continuously. And yet, despite my hopes to the contrary, running was not getting much easier. Stepping out the door was always a test of willpower; I still wore a fleshy coat, the night was a muggy sauna, and (at least half the time) I had spent the day with an empty stomach. Often, I would be completely spent at the end of my run, none too coherent but deliriously happy because I now had a full day to enjoy before my next run.

In early August, my athletic aspirations got a boost with the beginning of the 2002 World Cup. As a huge soccer fan (once literally, now only figuratively), I had World Cup fever. I was glued to the TV, even though the games took place in Korea and Japan, and matches aired between 3:00 and 9:00 in the morning on the East Coast. Team USA made a deep run into the tournament, and I leveraged my enthusiasm into my own workouts. In the four weeks of the tournament, I lost another eighteen pounds and another clothing size with them. One day, while casting about for a shirt that wasn't too big, I found a blue jersey that fit perfectly. Only after slipping it off did I realize that I had just fit into my old soccer jersey... from when I was twelve years old.

What's a major life change if you can't have a little fun along the way? People who saw me around work had long since noticed I was losing some serious weight. One of the secretaries was particularly fascinated. She hadn't been privy to my day-to-day struggles, and so (like many people) she thought I had some sort of special technique for effortlessly losing weight. Repeatedly, she approached me to find out what my secret was. I always told her that I was just working hard and eating right, trying to spare her the peculiarities of my experiment. Still she didn't believe me, jokingly telling me that she would discover my secret if it killed her.

Around this time, my research group had taken to ordering a large quantity of fried chicken for a group lunch every Friday. As low man on the totem pole, I was tasked with driving to KFC to collect our order, even though I often couldn't eat what I picked up. The same inquisitive secretary had a desk by the elevator, and she saw me time and again carrying several large buckets of fried chicken into our break room. Assuming all of this was for me, she came to the erroneous conclusion that I had discovered a secret diet allowing me to eat anything I wanted. One Friday, I was cleaning up the remains of the food from our meeting when she trapped me. This was a non-fasting day, and I had the last piece of chicken stuck in my mouth as I picked up the remains of enough food for six people. Seeing me in this compromising position only confirmed her suspicions. She decided to confront me.

"I knew it. I knew you had a secret to losing all that weight! It's the chicken, isn't it?" she asked excitedly.

Caught red-handed, I decided to play along and have a little fun with her. I confessed, telling her that the real secret to my weight loss was a diet consisting exclusively of fried chicken. I gave her particulars: All I was eating was original recipe fried chicken, no hot wings and no chicken strips. All chicken was to be eaten only with approved side items. Cornbread was OK, as was the mac and cheese; the rolls and mashed potatoes were forbidden. "Stay away from the pie," I concluded, tipping her an exaggerated, knowing wink. "It's the worst thing for you when you're on the chicken. That's what I call it. 'On the chicken.'" She nodded solemnly, committing every word to memory. I think I even saw her take a note or two.

A few days later, I was minding my own business, having forgotten the encounter, when the secretary appeared again with her cousin in tow. He was a chunky lad who, she explained to me, was also looking to lose weight.

"Noah, you gotta tell Devon about going 'on the chicken.' He wants to lose weight and he *loves* chicken," she said, gazing at me expectantly.

My inner thespian failed me; there was no way I could actually tell someone to go on an all-chicken diet with a straight face. In a flash, I had a plan that would keep them safe from my imaginary diet forever.

"Devon, your aunt didn't tell you the full story," I said ominously. "Before you get to the all-chicken phase, you have to prepare your body with the all-gizzard purification phase. It's really just like the Atkins diet...only with gizzards. For a month."

# The Delusional State of the Merely Big-Boned

*Self-delusion is pulling in your stomach*
*when you step on the scales.*

—PAUL SWEENEY

When August rolled around, it was time to begin packing for my move to Florida. As I gathered my possessions, it seemed prudent to also take a summary of my progress. By any measure, my diet had been wildly successful. I had been eating only every other day for a period of almost six months and exercising regularly for four of those. In that time, my weight had dropped from 341 pounds to 235—a loss of 116 pounds, or, in non-metrical terms, slightly less than two first graders. My dimensions had shrunk accordingly: my waistline had dwindled from 48 inches to 38, and I had abbreviated my XXL shirt tags to read merely L. I could now run distances measured in miles and minutes, as opposed to yards and seconds. Even my feet had slimmed down, as I had dropped from a size 16 to a 15. Most important, life was good again. I would get out of bed each morning refreshed and ready to face my life. By any measure, I was happy.

If there was any problem resulting from my rapid weight loss, it was that my body had beaten my mind to being thinner. Reading a scale and weight-range charts, I could see that I was now just a few pounds overweight by objective standards. This was clear, and yet I still thought of myself as huge. Sometimes I would dream that I was still fat and wake up in an agitated state. I couldn't really complain about how quickly my diet had worked, but a slower loss of weight would have allowed my mind to keep pace with the changes in my body and made it a little easier to answer the next question: What do I do now?

This was a complicated issue. Even though I had accomplished a great deal on the strength of my own wits and planning, I had no idea what to do once I fell into a normal weight range. For one thing, my perceptions of weight and health were still clouded. As I've said, no one grows to the proportions I reached without having a serious blind spot for the implications and problems (health-related and social) associated with increasing weight. Only now was I able to see how I had managed to deny the obvious. I had become adept at convincing myself that I wasn't really that out of shape. For example, I would be watching a football game on TV, and an announcer would mention that one of the offensive linemen was 6'5" and 340 pounds. I would think to myself something along the lines of *OK, look at that guy. He's the same height and weight as I am, and he's a professional athlete! Sure, he's probably in a little better shape than I am, but if we're the same exact size, I can't truly be that out of shape, can I?* Obviously, this was stretching it. For one thing, the football player had fifty or more pounds of pure muscle than I did, which makes a huge difference in body mass and composition. Second, the football player was still overweight, by no means necessarily in perfect health.[9] Third, not all professional athletes' body types are ideal for the average person to emulate. I was guilty of something of a logical fallacy by believing that two things were similar when, in fact, they were not.

This was by no means the only way I deluded myself. I turned a blind eye to my physical limitations, avoided opportunities to do physical activities in public, and (of course) shunned the scale, so as to have plausible deniability of the existence of a problem. Even now that I've addressed the problem, I remain ashamed of this blindness that allowed me to waste years of my life and consumed untold amounts of energy in covering up reality. There's an old joke among psychologists: most people have delusions of grandeur; I was having delusions of adequacy.

Like my self-perception, my estimation of what was an ideal, healthy weight was markedly skewed. Recall that, after realizing I was making real progress in my diet, I set a goal weight of 250 pounds. Why 250 pounds? To me, this sounded like a nice, healthy number to aim for. By the end of summer I weighed far less than this, and I still thought that I needed to shed a few more pounds to reach an ideal weight. Clearly, my perceptions of what was healthy changed as I lost weight. There was no knowing that a goal I set today would be appropriate tomorrow. Realizing this prompted a deeper question: How would I know when I'd completed my experiment? Would there ever be a point where I could say, "That's it. I've done what I set out to accomplish"?

The meanings of terms like "healthy" and "fit" were clearly relativistic and are frequently based on personal perception. When I first started to run, I could go for about two minutes before having to stop. Over a few months I had worked my way up to about half an hour of continuous running. I also knew I was also running a little faster, but was I really fit? Late in the summer, I got to run on a track and, for the first time ever, I clocked my speed. Going as fast as I could, I ran two miles at about 9:45/mile, a decent clip by recreational standards. But later that night, I wondered how my times stacked up against "real" runners. I called up the results from the previous year's New York Marathon. The winner had run almost exactly twice as fast as I did…for more than twenty-six miles! I scrolled down and saw that someone who ran at my pace would have finished in 13,500th place. And I could only keep it up for two miles! Though I had made tremendous progress in my own abilities, it was clear that the human body, generally speaking, was capable of much more.

It had also become apparent that many of my notions about health and fitness were somewhat antiquated. Above all, I had imagined that weight and fitness were inextricably linked, while in fact the two are only casually related. While there are clearly defined "healthy" ranges of weight and body composition, fitness is dynamic. I would soon have completed the challenge of reaching a normal weight. With that issue tabled, I was curious to discover just how far my athletic capabilities could be expanded. Undoubtedly, there remained much room for improvement. I was beginning to ask questions with no obvious answers: To what degree could the consequences of lifelong obesity be reversed? How much farther or faster could I go? How much could I change for the better?

I had no idea. But I really wanted to find out.

On my last day of work at Duke, there was a department-wide goodbye party in my honor. As luck would have it, the event was held on a day when I wasn't eating, so I couldn't partake of my farewell cake. During the course of the party, my fasting became a point of conversation; people throughout the building had noticed that I was rapidly shrinking and were curious about how I was doing it. The conversation turned into an impromptu lecture, as I explained to the crowd of mostly scientists the study on which I'd based my diet, described my addition of an exercise program, and quantified the dramatic results I had achieved. Most people were stunned by my odd approach, but they took no issue with my unorthodox methodologies and were generally very positive about the results. Only two of the thirty people in the room expressed any concern that what I was doing might not be so great. Coincidentally, they were also the only two people out of the group who might be considered obese.

"Don't you think starving yourself all the time is bad for you?" one of the two asked, her sentiments quickly echoed by her portly companion. There was no animosity or jealousy in her tone, only legitimate concern. It was somewhat hard for me to believe the question was serious, given who was asking it. I looked at them, trying to figure out how to answer. The girls were standing there, posing their queries between mouthfuls of the frosted cake I had eschewed. I knew instantly what I wanted to say, but I held my tongue for a moment. My reply was likely to offend them both. *To hell with it*, I decided. They could use a dose of the truth.

"I'm pretty sure being massively overweight is a hell of a lot more dangerous than just about any type of diet," I said. As I'd anticipated, the remark hit a little too close to home for the questioner, who winced slightly and, red-faced, excused herself, companion in tow, shortly thereafter. It didn't make sense to me why, of all people, someone with a weight problem would have said such a thing. Clearly, I was doing OK and had made a lot of progress. What could they possibly be concerned about?

A little later, the party broke up and it was time for me to make my departure. I boxed up my stuff and hopped on the bus for a ride across campus. Since I had taken to running at night now, I was in the habit of taking the bus from time to time and was on friendly terms with most of the bus drivers. The driver covering the afternoon shift for my bus route was both extremely gregarious and extremely large. Like everyone else, he had noticed the winnowing of my physique, and he had given me offhanded compliments about it over the course of the summer. As I was the only one riding the bus that afternoon, he unwittingly picked my final day to strike up a conversation. Like the secretary who thought I had some secret method, he wanted to know just how I managed to lose weight so quickly. He had a particular reason for his curiosity: he was thinking about going on a diet himself, and was looking for some pointers to get started.

This was the first time anyone had ever asked me directly for practical advice on losing weight. Thrilled that I might be inspiring someone to lose weight, I launched into an enthusiastic lecture on the effectiveness of intermittent fasting and exercise. As I was building momentum, the bus driver abruptly interrupted me and began a rambling diatribe about a previous failed attempt to diet. It was a familiar tale: he would start working out and eating right, but always wound up on the couch with a bag of potato chips. The point of his interruption wasn't really clear to me. Why was he talking about what didn't work, instead of listening to someone who seemed to know what did? Minutes passed as I listened to his problems. Suddenly, I found that I had gotten off at my stop and was left standing in a cloud of hot exhaust, watching the bus drive away. What the hell had just happened? I had communicated remarkably little information to the bus driver, and I wondered if he had gotten any benefit out of our interaction. Was I not doing a good job of answering his questions?

An explanation finally dawned on me. There *was* a definite reason for our one-way discussion, and the bus driver *had* gotten something out of it. The bus driver didn't really want to lose weight in any meaningful way, and he certainly didn't want to talk about the practicalities of actually doing so. He wasn't looking for advice or information. He was looking for peace of mind. The point of our talk was not for me to inspire him, but for him to explain how he'd tried to lose weight. He wanted to explain away his failures. Why would he waste his time doing that? What good is talking about something you have no intention of actually doing? And why would a person bother trying to justify a failed weight-loss attempt to someone who had succeeded?

In fact, I understood this behavior especially well. Not long ago, I had been equivocating about my own weight. I was well aware that if you're not willing to make a difficult change, the next best thing to do is to convince yourself and others that you tried your best to do so.

Nobility in failure, or something like that. If you can convince yourself that you've given your best effort, you can feel better about your lack of progress. What's more, if you can sell this argument to someone who's done what you've failed to do, you can rest easy with the satisfaction that your shortcomings have been validated and absolved by someone who is, at least in this regard, superior to you. *That* was the real point of the bus driver's story. Only recently had I become sensitive to my own rationalizing behaviors, and this was really the first time I had observed them in a stranger. To be frank, the sight was both horrifying and pathetic. From where I sat, all this bloviation was in service of a moot point. Regardless of the reason, the bus driver was still big.

There were obvious parallels between this encounter and my conversation with the overweight girls at the party. Both the bus driver and the girls were confronted by a person who had conquered a problem they knew they had failed to deal with. In the face of this knowledge, they sought to validate themselves, using different methods. Whereas the bus driver decided to rationalize his failure to me, the girls employed the tactic of minimizing my efforts. By questioning my diet's safety, the girls were able to attach a mental asterisk to everything I said. *It may have worked for this guy, but this weight-loss program isn't for me.*

The bus driver and the partygoers weren't searching for reasons to change, only excuses not to. By successfully losing weight, I was providing a living demonstration to these other heavy people that it was possible to get in shape. Confronted with the knowledge that another person had managed to conquer the obstacles they still faced, they were reminded of the choice in their hands: to do something about their weight, or to do nothing. Excuses, in their varied and extravagant form, are the decoration of those selecting the latter.

These two incidents were the first in a long series of similar encounters. It was as though I were some sort of priest, with a series of portly parishioners giving me confession as to why they chose not to lose weight. The excuses varied widely, but generally rested on the same basic tenets: it was never the fault of the individual, and there was usually an excellent reason why they couldn't do what I was doing (this was generally some variation on being too busy, typically with unspecified obligations). This paralogia was a trait shared by almost every heavy person I met, a sort of fattest common denominator. Confronted with so much self-deception, I began to file away the experiences, hoping to eventually explore just *why* people are willing to go to such lengths to shield themselves from something so physically and emotionally unpleasant as the realities of being overweight, rather than directly confronting and dealing with the problem. Of course, few people have the ability to realize that their rationalizations and equivocations are not valid reasons for avoiding an unpleasant issue. We all can go to great lengths to establish a reality that not only insulates us from the cold truth, but even shields us from our own moral compass when our instincts tell us what we're doing (or not doing) is wrong.

# It's Not the Heat,
# It's the Humidity

*Consult a physician before starting any
exercise plan. Cease exercising immediately
if you feel faint, dizzy, or experience pain or
shortness of breath.*

—WARNING ON A PIECE
OF EXERCISE EQUIPMENT

If I hadn't lost weight, I suspect I'd probably be dead now.

Not from a heart attack, stroke, high blood pressure, diabetes, or any
of the other usual culprits. Sure, I'd be heading toward all of them, but
they probably wouldn't have killed me by the time of this writing. I'm
talking about the heat in Florida. Going into the veritable furnace of
central Florida in August while carrying an extra hundred pounds of
fleshy insulation would have reduced me to a steaming pile of goo within days. I had a hard enough time as it was. I had bought a small house in
a development called Mile Run, a neighborhood I suspected was named
after the length of its central thoroughfare. The day after I moved in, my
father (still a paragon of fitness at fifty-five) took me on a little jog to test
this premise. It felt like we were running through a creamy bisque, the
air was so thick with humidity. When we'd finished, we paused a moment (giving me time to bend over double and wonder when exactly

I'd thought it was a good idea to move to Florida). As I struggled to live, several of my new neighbors spotted us and decided a neighborly southern introduction was in order. As the conversation dragged on interminably, I realized that I was going to either have to excuse myself to seek out air conditioning and fluids or pass out from dehydration. I carefully weighed the two options: showing physical weakness versus perpetrating social rudeness. A moment later I was hastily excusing myself and shuffling inside, to spend the next fifteen minutes lying on my kitchen floor, drinking directly from a gallon-sized water jug and listening to the faint sounds of my father explaining my sudden departure (something about me being Muslim and it being time for prayer). Fortunately, that was the only time I came close to passing out from the Florida heat. Unfortunately, it was the last time I ever spoke to those neighbors.

The creaking rustiness of my social skills was still quite fresh a few days later when I packed up the car again and headed south for a long awaited reunion with my girlfriend Jennifer. Jen had left North Carolina in April to pursue her dream job as a dolphin trainer in the Florida Keys, just as I began the first stages of dieting, and she hadn't been around to see any of the tangible results from my efforts. I had, of course, informed her of my progress over the phone, but she had not laid eyes on me in over four months. We had agreed to meet halfway, in the otherwise nondescript hamlet of Vero Beach. I picked out her car as soon as I pulled up, and she spotted me as I stepped out, weighing over a hundred pounds less than when she'd last seen me.

Have you ever seen someone completely and utterly shocked? If you're prepared for it, it can be quite comical. Jen did a double take and her eyes bugged out a little bit. Her jaw was working up and down, but no words were coming out. She blinked rapidly a few times (probably to make sure she wasn't seeing things), actually shook her head, and proceeded to express her surprise in terms not fit for print. She then went through the classic stages of grief in about three minutes: denial that this was actually me, anger at the loss of my chubby cheeks (her favorite of my previously rotund features), bargaining that she could accept the loss of the cheeks in exchange for not being accidentally squished while sleeping next to me, more depression over the loss of the chubby cheeks, and finally, acceptance that I weighed a whole lot less. Still, every few minutes, she would reach out to touch my now-tiny gut as if to assure herself that the flab was truly gone.

It was those kinds of reactions that made the effort worthwhile.

A few weeks later I started graduate school. On the first day I encountered another new experience since losing weight: I was accused of identity theft … of myself. The initial event of orientation week was in-person registration at the graduate students office. My photo had been taken when I had come to campus for the interview weekend, likely so that professors could put a face to a name when discussing candidates for admission. Unbeknownst to me, this photo was also put into my file for identification purposes. This seemed efficient enough, but for the small fact that I interviewed before losing weight, and now I no longer resembled the person in the photograph. As a result, I was apparently unrecognizable to the woman in charge of the check-in. As I told her my name, her eyes alternated from my face to the jowly picture of the person who had interviewed.

"You need to get your friend to come in and do this himself," she said, pushing aside my paperwork.

"Excuse me?" I asked, unsure of her meaning.

"I said you can't register someone else. Tell Noah he needs to come in and register himself. Now what's *your* name?" She began to re-scan the sheet of smiling faces, searching for the picture of the person standing before her.

"Noah Walton. I can spell it if you like."

She wasn't buying it. "Don't give me that. This," she stabbed my picture with her finger and glanced around cautiously to make certain that Noah wouldn't overhear, "…is a fat guy."

"*Was* a fat guy," I said, showing her my driver's license. Her eyes widened in surprise, but without embarrassment. "I'll be! You look great! Did you get gastric bypass or something?"

While graduate school was more than a little different from college (for starters, I had fifty classmates, as opposed to fifteen hundred), it nevertheless marked my return to an academic setting after more than a year. Though I loved the changes that I had produced in my life, I remained significantly insecure and understandably apprehensive about running into the same social stigmatization I had encountered in the previous phase of my education. I really didn't think I could spend another five or more years (in 2005, the average finishing time for a Ph.D. was a whopping 8.2 years)[10] in a state of more-or-less total social isolation.

The first weeks of my program were to be spent in a training laboratory, where we would work in teams to perform various types of experiments designed to acclimate us to the techniques we would employ as independent researchers. Shortly before the lab course started, there was a lunch for entering graduate students to let us meet one another. I thought this would be a grand opportunity to test how people who had never met me would react to me now that I was thinner. Naturally, I decided to start with the ladies. I plopped myself down in front of the cutest girl I could find, made a bit of small talk, and suggested that we work as lab partners.

My experiment yielded prompt results. Five years too late, I had confirmation of what I had long suspected: the skinny guys get all the girls. At least in the lab.

A week after school started, I had my first official soccer practice for the Gainesville city league. I'd talked my way onto a team over the summer, convincing the captain that I'd be a valuable player on the strength of my youth soccer experience and the fact that my registration check cleared. We did a few drills and I realized quickly that I was bad. Really bad. Bad to the point that I was lucky they didn't give me my money back at the end of the day. My triumphant return to soccer was marred by my utter lack of skill.

My soccer handicaps were in partly genetic. I possessed genes that were not wired for speed or coordination. As a child, I was noted for my exceptional lack of velocity, earning the charming nickname No-Motion-Noah in my first peewee soccer match. In addition, there was the matter of having spent the previous ten years with a giant gut hanging off of me. I had become accustomed to balancing myself while moving around like a fat person. My body clung to muscle memory and stubbornly refused to adapt to the fact that I was now substantially slimmer and (theoretically) more agile. My brain still thought I was huge, and it was reluctant to let me attempt maneuvers that would likely have hospitalized me some six months earlier. I was neuromuscularly ill-adapted to take advantage of the fact that I *could* move my arms and legs faster now that they carried less weight. Worst of all, my fat-man waddle was really, really slow. My running style was described by friends as resembling "a man riding a unicycle"—in essence, an unstable, tottering gait with a pronounced lurch. This evidence suggested that I might have permanently altered, possibly limited, my native physiological capacities by spending so many years overweight.

I continued to play soccer for many years for recreation and enjoyment, as part of a team formed by my classmates. My position on the roster was safe, as I formed close friendships with the team leaders that prevented me from being unceremoniously dumped in favor of better talent. Still, I remained concerned with my physical failings. I had predicated my experiment on the idea that I would find a way to push myself to a high level of physical excellence. But in what arena? With the limited physical abilities I possessed, demonstrating the mind-over-matter aspect of my hypothesis seemed that it would prove more challenging than anticipated.

# Lord, Deliver Unto Us... Pizza

*Use wisely your power of choice.*

—OG MANDINO

About a month after I started graduate school I was still shedding weight, albeit more slowly, and was down to about 225 pounds, a much more typical weight for my height. I decided that it was time to go off the intermittent fasting diet. This was a practical adaptation that needed to be made in light of my newfound enthusiasm for athletics. After working out seven days a week for five months straight, I had developed enough stamina to complete workouts I was unable to envision when I began. While I could now sustain a heightened level of cardiovascular activity, it was difficult to do so on an empty stomach. But abandoning my diet was like saying goodbye to an old friend. I thought about it for a few days, not ready to easily cast aside what had worked so well for me. And then one fasting morning, I was hungry, so I ate a banana. Just like that, the major weight-loss phase of my new lifestyle was over. It was anticlimactic. But I had never intended to spend the rest of my life eating only 50 percent of the time. It was time to learn how to maintain the healthy body I had worked hard to create. Proper daily nutrition would be my new challenge.

Ironically, having fewer rules requires even more self-control. Even while intermittently fasting, the days when I could eat were actually harder. On a fasting day, I thought of myself as being "on duty." The diet decisions were straightforward, written in stone, and easy to follow. On days without rules, I was almost lost from a complete lack of instruction—it was all about doing the right thing when no one was looking. I could eat whatever I desired, but did I really want to test how much my stomach could hold, knowing that I'd have to deal with the consequences tomorrow? Decisions to (even slightly) hold back on free days did just as much good as eating nothing on fasting days. Gradually introducing voluntary moderation in combination with involuntary rules in this manner was critical to producing a dividend from my diet and was the beginning of learning to make good eating decisions. Moderation in consumption was also important in aiding a physiological adaptation every dieter needs to make: by not gorging myself, I was not regularly stretching my stomach, and so I allowed it to shrink to hold (and feel full on) human-sized portions.

By leaving my alternate fasting rules behind, I was placing the decisions about when and what I ate wholly at my own discretion. This was akin to being released from prison on probation; I experienced both the uplifting and confounding aspects of being awash in freedoms. As for a parolee, the smart thing for me to do was buckle down, keep doing what worked, and avoid relapsing into the behaviors that had put me in a jam. Sometimes people don't make the right decisions, even when they're the obvious ones. I am sad to say that I didn't handle my newfound liberties well.

Despite twenty-two years of formal education, I was still painfully unprepared to live on my own, and I'd retained many of the feckless domestic habits common among college students. At the same time, I'd joined the department of neurobiology and was working long hours in the lab, studying the behaviors of neural stem cells. Often, I would arrive home exhausted, too unmotivated to do anything more than thumb through a take-out menu, much less cook. Trips to the grocery store were merely for gathering snack food; meals would come from whoever could find my house in thirty minutes or less. Pizza quickly became my new favorite food. Here's how bad it got: the guy who answered the phone at Papa John's had my credit card number memorized. At least four times a week I would call to order their perpetual special: a large pizza with a side order of greasy chicken strips with ranch dressing, and a two-liter bottle of Mr. Pibb (the surly southern relation of Dr. Pepper). At this point, I lived alone and had no one to help me finish this massive amount of food (or at least make me feel guilty for doing so myself). Invariably, food would arrive in the evening, and the next morning I would be finishing the last two slices of pizza and the remains of the soda for breakfast as I drove to the medical center. Like a misbegotten trollop in a Christian soap opera, I had lost my way.

From the sheer awfulness of my diet, it logically follows that I had no chance of maintaining a normal weight, and a huge backslide would accompany my actions. Indeed, I was trying to see what I could and couldn't eat now. I remained vigilant with the scale, prepared to re-embrace dietary martial law at the first sign of weight gain. A slide actually would have been helpful in keeping me on track, but surprisingly, it never materialized. I didn't gain any weight back. Not even an ounce. What resulted was a state of nutritional malaise; I was eating terribly, by any objective standard—and I knew it—but was doing nothing to change simply because I was getting away with it.

The only reason this spate of poor eating failed to trigger an explosion of my waistline was the fact that I was exercising more than ever. Since I had gotten myself down to a reasonable weight, I was able to play (albeit often poorly) any sport I wished. I longed to make up for time lost as an undergraduate, and the University of Florida was an ideal playground, a Mecca for pickup games and intramural sports. Some days I would play pick-up soccer, go home and eat various fried objects for dinner, and then go back to the gym and play basketball until the rec center closed. All of this activity was new to my body, and it was causing me to run hot. My metabolism was going a zillion miles an hour, effectively burning through all of the junk calories I was consuming. Still, even with this high level of activity, I ceased to lose any more weight, an indicator that my system was not perfect.

It's easy to cringe now at the number of empty calories I ate during that period. I felt disgusting after every meal, but I kept ordering the same food because it tasted good. Even though I looked OK, I began to experience the same feelings of low self-worth that had brought about my previous crisis of conscience.[11] While it was possible to imagine that I was merely taking a sort of vacation from the rigors of a long-term diet (and that is a dangerous thought for a recovering fatty, wouldn't you agree?), it became increasingly apparent that I was redeveloping my old habits, and fast. I became sickened, not with myself per se, but with my lack of discipline, and found more and more motivation to begin getting healthy again. I realized I had been lulled into a false sense of security by scale watching. Clearly there were better measures of what constituted health than the simple quantity of my weight. The challenge of finding fitness was more complicated now that number on the scale had ceased to be the all-important indicator.

Despite my recidivism, I was generally happy with my life. I had figured out a way to eat what I wanted while simultaneously avoiding gaining weight, and that felt good. Once again, it would have been easy to walk away from the remaining goal of my project, achieving excellence in an athletic discipline. After all, I reasoned, I'd already accomplished more than most people ever would. But I couldn't quit, even though I was ahead. It was impossible to justify abandoning my goal of becoming an elite athlete when I had barely gotten started. After all, my pursuit of that goal had gotten me to this point, and I felt as though I owed it to myself to follow through. Now the question was how to get my act together and resume my positive course.

While vigorous exercise had masked the deleterious effects of the poor dietary choices I had made, it had done me far more good than ill. Initially, I had used running to jumpstart my stalled weight loss, and now I hoped I could use it again to rescue myself from the doldrums in which I currently wallowed. Since I had come to Florida, I had largely abandoned distance running in favor of team sports that were more fun to play. Now I made the decision to re-emphasize running for the same reasons that I had been avoiding it. Pure running was a more demanding sport than my other activities and, because of this, was an extremely unpleasant experience when undertaken under the influence of dubious nutrition. My rationale was that I would *have* to clean up my diet to support the demands of being a runner. My initial goal was manageable: three runs a week, for a minimum of thirty minutes each. Nothing drastic; turning my life upside down again didn't seem to be in my best interest, as the combined stress of grad school and more hard dieting would derail me for certain. To this end, I made only one other change to my life. In a compromise between running-induced heartburn and my love for a forbidden fruit, I cut back the pizza ordering to once a week.

For a few months, I stuck with the minor changes I had made. I was rusty, as the team sports I'd been playing rarely required running over a hundred yards at a time. My long-distance running endurance was largely neglected and had suffered accordingly. I built back up to running four miles at a clip with a minimum of difficulty. Cleaning up my diet was surprisingly easy; in comparison to the draconian measures I'd taken in the past, it felt as though I had barely changed anything. I cut out the worst of my junk food binges and tried to eat a healthy lunch each day. Even with these modest efforts, I started to see results. I lost ten more pounds and, more importantly, felt great again. People who had only known me since I moved to Florida were now asking me if I'd lost weight, which made me smile even more.

The idea of running in a race occurred to me in late November. At first I was hesitant. Psychologically scarred from adverse conditioning, I found the notion of making a spectacle of myself none too appealing. Soccer was more my style; it gave me somewhere to hide when I was having a bad day, and I was reasonably certain that sitting on the bench when you got tired was not an option during a footrace. Actually, I'd barely even seen a road race before, and I was the sort of person who preferred to look before I leaped. The last time I'd tried something new athletically, ski patrol had to pull me off a mountain with a hyperextended knee. Nor was an injury the worst that could happen: with long-cultured athletic pessimism, I worried that I might finish last. Nevertheless, my curiosity was powerful. In December, a few of my classmates decided to run in a local 5K race for charity, one of those ubiquitous "Jingle Bell Runs" that crop up around Christmastime, and I allowed myself to be peer-pressured into joining them.

This race was as local as it got. The course was a loop through the campus of the University of Florida, with the starting line only a few hundred yards from my laboratory. Since it was being held on a weeknight, I needed only to change into running shorts and amble over after work. Not knowing any better, I played it safe and arrived about two hours early to check things out. I lurked around, sizing up the arriving runners and preparing to bolt early if it appeared I was going to be humiliated. Enough normal-looking people turned up to allay my concerns that I was going to finish last, but what really sold me were the jingle bells they were giving to participants to wear on their shoes. I declined the bells (so as not to draw unnecessary attention to myself), but the whole affair seemed low-key enough for me to pay a volunteer registration worker twenty bucks and head for the starting line.

I should mention at this point that I knew nothing about how to prepare for a race. I did no fancy (or even basic) training for it, no pre-race carbo-loading, nothing. I stretched, but had not done any warm-up jogging, as I was under the impression that it would only serve to tire me out and make me run slower during the actual race. I also had no notion of how tackle the race itself. The concept of pacing myself was largely foreign to me. The only advice I had gotten came from an eleventh-hour telephone call from my father, who told me not to start too fast. *No problem there,* I thought, as I seeded myself far back from the lean, greyhound-type runners who jockeyed for placement in the front rank. After an interminable pause, the gun went off and I charged forward ... directly into the person in front of me. Apparently it takes a moment or two for the runners in the back to get moving.

The traffic jam cleared quickly, and I had the presence of mind to start my watch as I crossed the start line. The course began by going downhill, and the favorable terrain turned the first half-mile into a merry sprint. Despite my conservative seeding before the start, I was being passed by anything on two legs. It had not occurred to me that other inexperienced runners often get caught up in the excitement and run too quickly early on, only to melt down toward the end. As it was, each person who passed was a blow to my fragile ego, bringing me closer to attaining the dubious distinction of race anchorman (a term I made up for the last official finisher).

I learned the difference between running for fun and running for competition right away. When you're out for a Sunday jog, you have normal thoughts and generally make rational decisions. When involved in organized competition, however, your mental capacity regresses to that of a high-strung six-year-old. Right now my inner first-grader was screaming one thing: *run faster!* I broke the glass and hit the panic button, increasing my pace to match those around me. In no time I was chuffing along in what could only be described as a panicky sprint-waddle, a prescription for speed my body could not hope to fill. Through the fog of the moment, my dad's advice to keep control reasserted itself, and I calmed down enough to maintain a nice, steady effort. Sure enough, I began passing tired people who weren't privy to the teachings of the elder Walton. The race flew by. The last quarter-mile was both tough and extraordinary. The racecourse looped back to the start line, and we finished by climbing the same hill we had run down to begin. The last few hundred yards went cross-country across an open field. Fighting painful hypoxia and sore legs, I passed a final knot of flagging racers to the approval of the gathered crowd.

As I caught my breath, I realized that this probably marked the first time a stranger had applauded a sports-related effort of mine. My first race was a lot like losing my virginity: it was over too quickly and I couldn't wait to do it again. I didn't even have to do well to enjoy myself—although I discovered I wasn't exactly terrible at running. I was amazed to find that I had easily avoided last place, coming in 108th out of 341 people, and had beaten my classmates for bragging rights in our program. Even though being the fastest graduate student in a biomedical research department was like being the tallest dwarf in the circus, this was one of only a handful of times that I had finished in the top half of ANY athletic competition. On the drive home, I was already wondering whether I could do better next time. Like a gambler on a hot streak, I didn't want to lose the feeling of doing so well.

My next opportunity turned out to be a few weeks later, when I traveled to North Carolina for winter break. My father, no doubt pleased with my blossoming interest in his favorite sport, challenged me to another five-kilometer race on New Year's Day for family bragging rights. I accepted the challenge. The father-son showdown was an interesting match-up: I was twenty-three but a relatively novice runner, whereas my father was three decades older but a veteran of countless running races. We spent the week of Christmas running together, sizing each other up, and talking trash. It was classic: old age and wiliness pitted against youth and inexperience. And there was treachery in spades. The night before the race, my father employed one of the dirtiest tricks I have ever witnessed. On New Year's Eve, he convinced me to accompany him to the local Outback Steakhouse, where he goaded me into ordering a Bloomin' Onion and the fettuccine alfredo. He watched me wolf these down from behind a plate of grilled salmon and steamed vegetables. I was about to learn a valuable lesson on proper pre-race nutrition. As I dozed off that night in the throes of a powerful food coma, I wondered just what my father had been chuckling about on the car ride home from the restaurant.

The next morning we drove to Raleigh for the big event. The race-course was a little more than three miles, like my first. As a veteran of exactly one race, and without being able to rely on my father to help plan strategy, I had formed my own battle plan. My intentions were to shadow my father for the first mile then make a move on one of the course's many hills. I would try to get a little lead, and then hope to hell he faded. Early on, all went according to plan: my father set the pace, and I stayed on his shoulder, ready to pounce. Shortly before the first mile marker I made my move. I surged ahead and opened a small gap, but my father doggedly stuck with me. My father is over a foot shorter and fifty pounds lighter than I, which must have made the two of us look, to the casual observer, like a graying David chasing after Goliath. At mile two I was still holding the lead. I was preparing a final surge to break away when a crippling pain savaged my insides. I felt as though someone had begun to operate a jackhammer in my colon. The previous evening's meal had apparently finished its tour of my digestive tract and was now ready to move on. I had a choice: slow my pace or soil my pants. I made the classy decision. Ten seconds later, my father made his final pass. Though he denies it to this day, I could have sworn I heard another chuckle as he went by. In the end, he beat me by about thirty seconds, then watched as I ran across the line and directly into a port-o-potty. When I emerged, I was pleased to discover that, while I was now the running "feeb" of the family, I had bested my time from two weeks ago by over two minutes and finished in 56th place. I vowed that the next time my father wouldn't be so lucky.

Unfortunately, I never got the chance to claim the family running title. The New Year's Day 5K of 2003 turned out to be the penultimate race of my father's career. A bad hip forced him to get surgery, and his doctor advised him to avoid running, killing any chance I had at vengeance. Thwarted as I was by this unfortunate condition, my father's bad hip wasn't quite done with me—it would re-enter my life in just a few short months.

# Gastric Bypass

*It puts the lotion on its skin.*
*Or else it gets the hose again.*

—BUFFALO BILL,
*SILENCE OF THE LAMBS*

One day, while watching TV, I came across a show about people who underwent surgical interventions to prevent them from overeating. These procedures, usually referred to as gastric bypass (or, generically, bariatric surgery), involve limiting the size of the stomach and rerouting the digestive path past a section of the small intestine. With decreased stomach space for holding food, and less absorption of calories through the small intestine, overweight patients experienced dramatic initial weight loss, according to the show. At the time, bariatric surgery was being hailed as the hot new treatment for obesity. For the first time, I wondered why I hadn't seriously considered looking into one of these procedures for myself.

Before I had begun to diet, I had disregarded out of hand any kind of surgical intervention for weight loss. As mentioned, I had a tendency to minimize the severity of my problem, and seriously entertaining such a dramatic measure would have been tantamount to acknowledging how overwhelming things had become. I also suspect that my attitude toward the procedures were heavily influenced by my aversion to being flayed open by a stranger, a common occurrence in surgeries. As I began losing weight on my own, I came to believe that weight loss should be achieved by addressing and solving the problem on your own, so that the process would make you stronger. Using surgery to achieve the goal seemed like cheating: how can you truly know that you can live a healthy lifestyle if someone makes it impossible for you to overeat? And what would it say about you if you somehow managed to regain weight, despite having a stomach the size of an egg?

This last question has become unexpectedly pertinent, as gastric bypass becomes more established and tracking data on participants accumulates. A 2007 Swedish study,[12] among the first to track surgical patients for a full ten years, revealed some disturbing trends in weight loss. Typically, patients lost a significant amount of weight by the end of their first year; around 25 percent of their original bodyweight, on average. Certainly, this had something to do with patients literally not being able to consume an excess of calories with their new, tiny stomachs. However, in the following nine years, a disturbing trend developed. Rather than continuing to lose weight, patients experienced the opposite: they began to regain the weight they had lost immediately following the surgery. Ten years after undergoing surgery, the average participant had regained more than half of his total weight loss. Almost 10 percent of the patients had actually gone *above* their original weight in the same period of time. This is a troubling finding. It demonstrates that people who fail to modify their poor eating behaviors over time are doomed to fail at losing weight, even when their poor behaviors are restricted by a fairly significant surgical procedure. The data also reaffirmed a belief I had that I had been incubating: no matter how hard you try, it's impossible to impose weight loss on a person who's not committed to the goal.

While weight-reduction surgeries were never my thing, I did investigate plastic surgery in the wake of my own weight loss. Most people who overcome severe obesity, especially those who lose weight quickly, as I did, are in a way victims of their own success. Since skin cells are rarely deliberately broken down by the body, there was little chance that the excess skin that was once necessary for the rolling expanse of my gut would ever go away. Folds of loose-hanging skin combined with de-stretched stretch marks are not a particularly flattering look for anyone, especially during beach season or shirts-and-skins football. The extra skin was definitely cramping my style, and it had to go. My mother, in a generous gesture, offered to pay for the necessary plastic surgery. And so, late in 2003, I made an appointment to see a surgeon in Washington, D.C.

My initial consultation was at the surgeon's office. While my mother and I waited, we chatted with the doctor's receptionist. She asked me what I was there for, and I briefly rehashed the story of my weight loss and explained that I was now looking to remove the excess skin from my torso.

"Oh, you got gastric bypass?" she asked casually. I told her I had lost the weight on my own. That got her attention. "Really? On your own? I can't remember the last person to come through the door who lost that much weight without surgery."

I was flattered, but a little taken aback. "I guess I'm not most people," was all I could manage in response.

Dr. Saeed Marefat would be performing my procedure. Like most medical doctors working in an often-touchy field, he was professionally clinical to the point of iciness. During the interview, he asked a standard battery of questions, including whether I'd had surgery of any kind. When I told him the greatest operation I'd endured was having my wisdom teeth removed, he raised an eyebrow. "Really? No gastric? That's not very common."

"That's what I hear," I said.

We settled on a procedure called a partial abdominoplasty. Dr. Marefat would begin with a slightly curved incision from one hipbone to another, creating a flap of flesh. The circumference of my belly button would be incised, freeing the skin and underlying tissue. Then the skin covering my torso would be raised off my abdomen and pulled downward, like a sheet, to overlap with the first flap. Once the skin was pulled taut, the excess flesh would be trimmed away and the remainder would be sutured back together. I would have a new belly button cut out, which would be re-anchored to where the old one was, and everything would be good as new. Two small liposuctions from my sides would complete the aesthetic effect. I would have a fourteen-inch scar curving between my hip bones, but it would be below my waist and thus invisible as long as I was wearing clothes.

The surgery was scheduled for December 30, so that the majority of my recovery period would fall during a break in school. While I was eager to part with one of the last reminders of my old body, my mother was also excited in anticipation of sequestering her only child for a full ten days. The night before the operation there was a cosmetic surgery show on the Discovery Channel. As luck would have it, the subject of the show was having almost exactly the same procedure I was about to undergo. After watching it in grim fascination, I belatedly decided that ignorance was bliss when it came to surgery. The major surgical incisions I was fine with. I was OK with the bedsheet-like skin-pulling action and with having a surgically manufactured belly button. What got to me was watching the liposuction. The surgeon was rooting around vigorously with a trocar just below the skin. It was like watching a chef inject butter under the skin of a chicken, only in this case I guess he was taking the butter out. Either way, I slept poorly that night.

The morning of the procedure, my simmering nervous energy was transformed into raw, naked apprehension, as I had realized that someone *was* going to be slicing me open after all. On the drive in, I gave my mother explicit instructions to sue the surgeon if I died, and specified how she should distribute the money from the settlement. I also stipulated that some of my ashes be inserted in a golf ball, which Tiger Woods would then drive into the Pacific Ocean. My mother nodded serenely, as though this was a normal request. In the pre-operative waiting room, the doctor drew a number of marks on my skin in ticklish places. Trying to break the tension, I asked him if it was possible to save the skin he would be paring away. He asked why. I told him I was hoping to make a pair of mittens and quoted him a few lines from *Silence of the Lambs*. He didn't smile.

As they laid me out on the table, the anesthesiologist made small talk while he administered the general anesthetic. "I see you're getting an abdominoplasty. Did you lose the weight as part of a gastric bypass program?"

"No, I lost all the weight on my own," I answered.

"You don't say!" he exclaimed. "We don't see much of that here."

My comeback was cut off by my loss of consciousness as the drugs kicked in.

I greatly enjoyed being anesthetized. It felt like the deepest, most satisfying sleep I'd ever gotten. Everything was right with the world, and all my troubles melted away. Slowly, gradually, I drifted back into reality as a nurse yelled at me to wake up.

My first order of business was making sure everything I'd wanted to keep was still there. I had been reading about surgical accidents and was quite concerned about having something other than unwanted skin accidentally removed. The morning before we left for the surgical clinic, I took the liberty of twist-tying a note to myself explaining what was and what was not to be excised. I attached the note to a part of me that I particularly didn't want to lose. When I woke up, the note was gone, but everything else was still there. And I noticed that all the nurses kept smiling at me.

While I was unconscious, someone had stuffed me into a tight-fitting compression girdle to remold the skin to my abdomen. I was told

I needed to wear it for everything but bathing for six weeks. I was stuck in this spandex wife-beater for six weeks!?! *Now they tell me.* I was given two girdles, one black and one white, presumably to equip me for both casual and formal functions. After all of this was explained to me, I was helped to my feet to head home. As I stood up to leave the operating room, I noticed three tubes coming out of me, each one attached to a little baggie filled with red fluid. "Excuse me," I asked the nearest health care professional. "Why are there tubes coming out of me?"

"Those? They're the drains from your incision. They'll come out in about a week," was the answer. No one had mentioned drains. This deal just kept getting better. At least none of the tubes was a catheter. A few minutes later, I shuffled out to the car accompanied by my entourage of tubes, pills, and specialized clothing.

My convalescence was not pleasant. The first day was OK, but then the really good pain medication wore off. Many times, I told my mother to go ahead and sue my doctor, not for negligent death, but for the wanton infliction of pain and suffering. To best sum up the experience to the uninitiated I say this: Have you ever heard older people who say they're willing to die rather than undergo another surgery? I understand them now. I am ashamed to say I lost the will to live within three days, but I was not sufficiently maimed to expire, so I was left in a purgatory of sorts. I learned a lot of things the hard way, the most important of which was that under no circumstances should a patient in my situation take a shower until the midsection is firmly healed. Each falling water droplet was like shrapnel to my tender, swollen skin. For the first few showers, I was dangerously close to enacting the "I've fallen, and I can't get up!" commercials. Equal to the pain, boredom was also a formidable obstacle to my recovery. Even sleeping was a substantial challenge, lest I accidentally flip to onto my stomach during the night. If it hadn't been for the college football bowl season and several thick Herman Wouk novels, I might not have made it.

But through it all, I got a little better each day. After a few days I realized I could walk without pain (or at least with no more pain than I felt when stationary), and I would go out and walk a few miles, tubes and all, just because it made me feel a little more human to be active again.

I learned that almost four pounds of skin were removed during the procedure. It took a long time to heal fully from the skin removal. The results were quite nice, although I permanently lost a bit of sensation near my belly button. Given the choice now, I would have the abdominoplasty all over again. But still, no gastric bypass for me. I could take recovering from one operation, but two was probably one too many.

# Going Long

*I know God will not give me anything I can't handle. I just wish He didn't trust me so much.*

—MOTHER TERESA

After much debate, I decided to make my way up in the world of running by trying my hand (and legs) at a longer race. If I was going to give running a serious try, it was incumbent on me to discover what kind of runner I was. I had learned that even something as simple and intuitive as running could be broken down into very distinct specialties. There are actually two major types of races: those catering to "fast" runners and those designed for "distance" runners. Fast runners excel at the briefer races, usually ranging from track meets to 5- and 10-kilometer races. These speedsters do best when giving their maximum effort over a relatively short period of time and racing at their speed threshold right from the gun. Long-distance specialists run races of 15 kilometers up to 26.2-mile full marathons. These runners rely on their capacity for steady, aerobic exercise, running far more strategically than the sprinters and parceling out their hardest efforts as tactical gambits.

A person makes many physical adaptations when specializing him- or herself for speed or distance running. To see this, one need only compare the tree-trunk legs of sprinters with the willowy frames of top marathoners. This is not to say that speed and distance are diametrically opposed, as the two worlds are closely related. Distance runners regularly practice running fast to build leg speed, and the speed demons will occasionally do long runs to build their endurance. I have met plenty of good recreational runners who were successful at both types of races, but even these versatile athletes usually had a preference when asked. At the elite level, specialization is the rule. Distance runners can be pretty fast, but even they rarely compete with their speedy counterparts over shorter distances, and vice versa. Naturally, I wanted to be as competitive as I could, and that would eventually involve finding my racing niche.

Like many great ideas, my plan to try longer races was born out of necessity. Specifically, I had an epiphany during a soccer game. A ball was played into open space, and I was forced to sprint at top speed to reach it. After reaching top speed (a lengthy process in itself), I realized that I was running so slowly I actually had time to think about how slowly I was running. A sarcastic little voice began playing through my head. *So... this is it, eh? Seriously? Any chance of going any faster? No? Might want to try something different there, partner, 'cause this ain't workin'.*

Always listen to the little voice.

Thus far, my competitive running experience had been in shorter, faster-paced races. I had not selected them because I considered myself predisposed to shorter distances, but because I considered myself physically incapable of running anything longer. As I began to cover more distance in my everyday runs, it became apparent that I was now physically able to complete the distances demanded in longer races. At this point, preoccupied with wondering where I should compete, I failed to think about whether I should even be running at all. This was probably fortuitous, as I had neither the background nor the body of a runner of any type. I lacked the leg speed and classic running form to be a really viable short-distance runner. Nor was I a prototypical distance runner; I was a foot taller than the average pro marathoner, and a good bit heavier to boot. Unaware that I was condemned to fail by the conventional wisdom of the running community, I decided to try distance running. As I saw it, I had three traits that predisposed me to this sort of running: the discipline to do the difficult training, a good tolerance for discomfort, and the willingness to craft a master strategy for success, something I particularly enjoyed doing. Not coincidentally, these were the same attributes that steered me to success in dieting.

To officially kick off my career as a distance runner, I signed up for the venerable Gate River Run in Jacksonville, Florida. It was a full 15K race, three times longer than the events I'd tackled previously. I had two months to prepare for it. Since there was little time to experiment, I set myself to learning what experienced runners and coaches recommended for conquering this distance. One of the few things everyone agreed upon was the need to build fitness by adding a longer run each week. Every Sunday I would do a single lengthy run, slowly increasing the distance from five miles to eleven miles—longer than the length of the actual race. The idea behind the long run was simple: get your body used to running for a long period of time. Between Sundays, I would do shorter runs at a slightly faster pace. Because I was running more miles than ever, my large frame had become a bit sparer, and I dropped a little more weight to reach a new low of 210 pounds before the race.

In the week before the race, my apprehension began to build. Once again, I was in uncharted territory. This was my first out-of-town race, and I had only recently discovered that the Gate River event had the added distinction of being the national championship race for the 15K distance. I would be participating in a race with some of the best runners in the world, a daunting prospect, particularly since I was already doubting my abilities. To further increase my apprehension, the course was the most challenging I had ever faced: rolling hills, with the final miles featuring a climb over the immense Hart Bridge, which spans the Intracoastal Waterway.

On race morning, the sheer size of the event caught me off guard. The biggest race I had run to date had slightly more than three hundred participants; Gate River had over seven thousand registered racers. I marveled at the egalitarian nature of running, such that someone like me could line up with (OK, behind) Olympic-quality runners and the current world champion at the 15K distance. Even though I was going to be firmly entrenched in the middle of the pack, the fact that this race was *the* national championship made me feel added pressure to perform. One extra trip to the port-o-potty later, I nestled into the sea of humanity as the starting cannon went off. In consideration of the distance and difficulty of the course, I held back in the early going and so reached the Hart Bridge in reasonably good shape. We made a left-hand turn and there it was, towering over us all. The bridge was everything it had been made out to be. *How the hell am I going to get to the top of that thing?* I wondered. I looked for, but was unable to find, a way around. It appeared I had no choice but to climb the beast. A group playing tribal drums had set themselves up at the base of the climb, possibly in an effort to help us imagine we were all preternaturally speedy African runners. Imagining myself as the largest, lightest-skinned man in the history of Kenya, I charged the bridge.

Allow me to state the obvious: running uphill is significantly more difficult and less pleasant than running on level ground. My legs felt as though they were encased in invisible shackles, and my pace slowed to little more than a glorified shuffle. My gaze was fixed on the summit of the bridge, which, maddeningly, did not appear to be getting any closer.

People occasionally ask me what I think about when I'm running. Shorter races happen so quickly that my mind has no time to wander, but on a longer jaunt like this one there is time to ruminate. At the moment, my thoughts dwelled on literature—specifically, whether the coppery taste in the back of my throat was the same taste of pennies and death that Hemingway describes in "The Snows of Kilimanjaro." Any

such sophisticated musings were soon drowned out by a far more pro-
saic sentiment: *Don't die, don't die, don't die.* I wasn't alone in this regard.
I passed another runner, listing dangerously and somehow moving even
more slowly than me, who muttered the single word "OhmyJesus!" on
each massive exhalation. After an eternity, we ran out of vertical real
estate. Reaching the apex of the bridge was bliss. For the first time in my
life, I was happy to say that there was nowhere to go but down. There
was more suffering and aching of legs, but I ultimately completed my
first long race in an hour and twenty-three minutes.

The finish line of a big race offers a tremendous sense of satisfaction.
The crowds of spectators at Gate River were concentrated in the last
half-mile, and I was picked up and carried on with energy I didn't think
I had. After I finished, the feedback I got from my body was absolutely
incredible. Crossing the line, I experienced the sensation referred to by
some as "runner's high." The sensation is a mixture of natural endor-
phins, extreme gratitude for surviving the experience, and happiness
over not having to run anymore.

Whether it was because of the gratification of finishing, the excitement of the race, or something else entirely, I was smitten with my new
pursuit. Long-distance running was comfortingly familiar, and I slipped
into it like something I was born to do. The experience of competing
in a hard, long race offered the same challenges and rewards of dieting, only in microcosm. Both take time to achieve, and both can be unpredictable experiences. There are times when you feel good and also
inevitable moments when you feel you need to quit. The perseverance
to overcome these moments was something I understood, and I felt a
certain familiarity with the mindset required by endurance sports. Indeed, my previous experiences were good place to start from. I decided
that, as long as I still felt the desire to compete, I would continue to run
long-distance races and strive to improve.

# Branching Out

*Lord! We know what we are,*
*but know not what we may be.*
—WILLIAM SHAKESPEARE

I raced twice more in 2004, both times in longer events, both resulting in new personal bests. My aims were still modest: I was mostly participating in small, local races, and while I wasn't a threat to win anything, I was moving my name up the results page. My improvement was rapid, and running began to feel more and more natural to me. Human beings have evolved to run, not quickly, but over long distances. Like most of our species, I found it almost unnatural to consider myself anything but the pinnacle of evolution; my estimation of my potential had gotten perhaps a bit too lofty. Fortunately, running was proving an excellent check for an overweening ego, and it kept me humble.

In my last race of the year, I lined myself up at the front of the field among the "real" runners. A third of the way into the race, a woman I had been leading drew alongside, matching my pace. She appeared to be lurching pretty badly, and my practiced eye identified several signs of a classic movement disorder. My best guess was multiple sclerosis, maybe early-onset Parkinson's. It looked like she was already struggling and was going to burn out long before the finish line, a common fate for inexperienced runners racing to raise money for charity. I leaned in and told her I thought it was just terrific that she didn't let her physical limi-

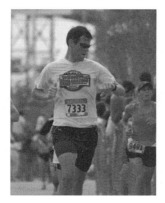

From the online edition of the Florida Times-Union, my second attempt at Gate River Run.

tations control her life. She gave me a funny look and didn't reply. Perhaps she didn't like talking about her disease.

At the halfway point, I realized that not only had this woman kept up with me, she was now outpacing me, and had begun to open a gap. It's important to mention here that I have no problem with being beaten by a woman. But this was different; I simply could not handle losing to someone with an advanced degenerative neurological condition.

*Noah to legs: more power!*

It wasn't working. I tried again. *Legs, I repeat: more speed!*

But it was to no avail. Gasping for breath, I was helpless to stop her from cruising away. In the end, she wound up beating me by more than three minutes. I finished the race, still a little confused. I had posted a solid time, and she'd beaten me fair and square. But how did she do it so easily? At the awards ceremony, the same woman was called to the stage. *Here's where they recognize her for fighting through her physical limitations,* I thought. It didn't quite go down that way. The news was mixed: on the upside, she didn't have a movement disorder. While my ego was temporarily salved by this revelation, there was also some bad news: the reason the woman moved so spastically was because she hadn't been running—she was an Olympic-level race walker! So while I remain (to my knowledge) undefeated by anyone in the late stages of a debilitating disease, I have once been outwalked.

In 2005 I ran the Gate River race for a second time, finishing more than eight minutes faster than the previous year. This was a testament to my growing comfort with distance running. While I was targeting progressively longer races, I was easing into each new distance slowly and exploring it before trying something more ambitious. I was trying to avoid the distance-runner stereotype of being obsessed with running longer races simply for the sake of bragging rights. Too often, runners rush their development, usually with the goal of running a marathon.

The marathon deserves special discussion as a widely recognized accomplishment. Although I'd yet to attempt one, I had come to the opinion that interest in running a marathon often comes from ego, rather than the desire to test oneself. In 1995, Oprah Winfrey ran the Marine Corps Marathon, triggering a second running boom in the United States that attracted a wave of new runners to the sport. Many of these newcomers were not actually interested in running per se, but wished to complete a marathon to cross it off their "life list" of things to do. As a result, the number of people competing in marathons surged, and many big city races have essentially transformed into parties with a running problem. Marathons in Chicago, New York, and Honolulu routinely boast more than 40,000 participants, with average finishing times more than an hour slower than in previous decades. The presence of runners ill prepared to run the distance was evident from the casualties suffered in the 2007 Chicago Marathon, where higher than normal temperatures resulted in a huge number of heat-related medical emergencies, and more than a quarter of the participants failed to finish.

The point of this history is to illustrate the consequences of what happens when a person is in love with the *idea* of running, not running itself. Participation in sports is fun, and a part of being healthy, but participation in distance running involves a substantial investment. Only after several years did I finally begin to appreciate the dedication and long-term commitment required by the sport. I didn't think I was better or more worthy than the casual runner, but my goals were different, and I was following a path that I noticed was likely to produce successful endurance athletes. Unlike the "marathon first" casual runner, runners who were competitive at longer distances, in my observation, rarely started with the marathon as their primary goal. In most cases, these individuals worked up to that distance, first running three- to five-mile cross-country races in high school, then intermediate distances such as the 10K. Oftentimes, successful marathoners emerge because they are ineffective at shorter distances (for example, they lack the finishing speed to win short races). While I had waited far longer in life to get started than the typical distance runner, I thought it was logical to recapitulate the normal developmental path in order to reach my full potential.

In the spring of 2005, fate conspired to make my burgeoning athletic career take a left-hand turn. My father, always my role model for endurance sports, was increasingly plagued by hip pain. A degenerating hip socket was the culprit, and it proved resistant to non-surgical remedies. One complete hip replacement later, Dad was more or less forced to hang up his running shoes. Never one to easily acquiesce to a sedentary lifestyle, he began the unenviable search for a pain-free source of regular exercise. From a short list of possibilities, he selected cycling, an activity whose predictable range of motion was conducive to the maintenance of his shiny titanium hip.

My father discovered he loved to ride, almost as much as he loved running. Soon he was on his bike almost every day, climbing the hills near his home in central North Carolina. At some point, he made the decision that I too should get into cycling. I suspect he missed running with me and was motivated by the desire for a cycling partner during my visits home. When he first broached the idea, I was skeptical. I hadn't ridden a bike in almost fifteen years, and I wasn't completely sure I even remembered how. What I did seem to recall was that cycling involved wearing spandex and shaving one's legs. One by one, my father wore my objections down and convinced me to try biking, largely on the strength of his offer to buy me a bike.

With someone else's money in hand, I spent a pleasant afternoon in May shopping for my new ride. I walked into the local bike shop not knowing the first thing about cycling culture. I didn't even know how to go about buying a bike. I was operating under the mistaken impression that bike shops were akin to car dealerships, where haggling over the price was a *de facto* part of the process. The manager of the shop walked over and I immediately began negotiating, making it clear that I would walk out that instant unless he was serious about cutting me a good deal. He looked at me like I was on drugs. After being gently educated, I told him I was a rookie and was looking for a bike that would let me figure out if riding was for me. He looked me up and down and wheeled over the biggest bike in the shop: an aluminum-framed Trek 1000. I regarded the bike with the same pensive facial expression worn by clueless men everywhere as they listen to their mechanic explain what's wrong with their car. I had no idea if this was a good bike, but it was the same brand Lance Armstrong rode, so how bad could it be? The store employees asked me if I'd like to take it for a test ride. I was tempted to say no, fearful that my rustiness would result in an ugly wreck in front of the cool guys hanging around the shop. Biting back my reservations, I took the bike out for a wobbly spin of maybe a mile. I still had absolutely no idea if the bike was any good or not. More pleased to have survived the demo than anything else, I bought the bike and arranged to pick it up the next day.

Though I'd gotten a bike, the need for basic accessories such as a lock, a tire pump, or even a helmet had slipped my mind. Not to worry: when I arrived home that day, I was greeted by a large box from an online cyclery store. My father had been busy shopping for me, and I was now fully outfitted. The following afternoon I returned to the bike shop with a helmet and a check and left with my new bike. I looked at the traffic thundering by, said a silent prayer, put a toe in the pedal strap and pushed off. It was barely eight miles from shop to home, but the trip was anything but easy. The major hazard to my health was my general inability to handle a "real" bike. The last bike I'd had was from China via Wal-Mart, weighed maybe forty pounds, and had fat, knobby tires and a fluorescent decal identifying it as the "Road Python." The sleek affair I was now precariously perched upon was half that weight, with impossibly skinny tires and steering far more responsive than what I was used to. I was zigging and zagging all over the road, instigating some close encounters with irritated motorists. Even after getting a handle on my directional issues, I was still distracted by other things. My bike was equipped with a computer that attached to the handlebars. It told me how fast I was going and had a timer and an odometer. In short, it was engrossing. I had to learn very quickly that if I kept watching the computer as though it was a TV, I was destined to become a traffic fatality.

Thirty minutes later I pedaled into my driveway, lost my forward momentum, and almost toppled off the saddle before getting a foot down. Even after only half an hour on the bike, I was in mortal fear for my butt. The seats on racing bicycles are narrow and pointy, and they do no favors for the unprotected gluteus maximus. To combat this, cyclists usually wear skintight shorts with a cushioning pad in the seat. I had received such a pair but was originally recalcitrant at the idea of strutting around in spandex. Mounting my new bike in cargo shorts and with a backside unaccustomed to riding meant that my bike's saddle felt like a prostate-pulverizing piston on each little bump in the road. With no additional prompting, I began working through my issues regarding the metrosexual appearance of spandex.

I wasn't completely sold on the life of a cyclist by the time I went out for my first real ride that weekend. My perception of the sport of cycling was that it wasn't very challenging compared to running and that it would detract from my efforts in that arena. Still, it was fashionable to cross-train, and I wasn't independent enough to buck that particular trend. I had to ask my father how far was a reasonable distance to ride,

and he advised me to try twenty-five to thirty miles to start. I decided
to ride to a nearby town called Alachua, about twelve miles away. I left
my house, going about twenty miles per hour, and still figuring out exactly how the gear shifters worked. As I'd suspected, it was really easy—
I was zipping along effortlessly. If this was all there was to riding a bike,
I might want to try the Tour de France later that year.

I got to Alachua with no trouble and turned around to come back,
only to collide with the immutable laws of classical physics. Unlike in
running, the speed and direction of the wind play a fairly significant
role in how fast you can go on a bike. There is increased air resistance
when you're traveling at higher speeds. Unbeknownst to me, a rather
stiff breeze had been at my back on the way to Alachua, and this had become a spicy little headwind for the return leg of the journey. My speed
dropped from twenty to twelve miles per hour— I was crawling along
so slowly I could see old gum stuck to the pavement. After what seemed
like half a day I made it back, managed to rack my bike, and crawled
to the couch to drink some Gatorade and eat a giant brownie. I took
back everything I'd thought about cycling being easy; I felt soreness in
muscles I didn't know I had. Cycling was very different from running,
but it was also hard, in its own way.

What they say about learning to ride a bicycle is at least partly true:
my skills *were* coming back to me as I continued to pedal around town.
In addition to adapting to the ergonomics of riding, I was starting to
enjoy certain other aspects of road cycling. Going fast on a summer
day provided a nice breeze, a welcome change from the often-stifling
humidity in Florida. Riding was also really good for taking a few more
pounds off, and the world certainly looked nicer from the saddle of a
bike than from the front seat of a car.

After a few months of cycling, I began to question whether it would
be a sport in which I could excel. Being a big guy, I could put out a good
bit of power, which meant I could motor along at a good clip. Even so,

many of the same problems I faced in running plagued me here. Competitive cycling involves frequent, explosive accelerations, something I did not excel at producing. Nor was I terribly adept at propelling my big body up long hills, a prerequisite for success at the higher levels of cycling. I seemed doomed as a single-sport athlete. Once again, another opportunity presented itself; upon learning of my dual passions for running and cycling, one of my sports-oriented friends mentioned that I might consider trying a triathlon. Though I had heard of triathlons, my response to the suggestion ("That's the one where you run, then ski, then shoot, right?") belied my ignorance. I was gently informed that a triathlon entailed swimming, biking, and running, and that I had apparently just made up a sport.

The idea of doing a triathlon incubated in my mind over a couple of months. The more I thought about it, the more reasons I could see why I might be good multiple-sport athlete. Biking in triathlons were far steadier efforts than in stand-alone cycling races, which suited to my existing cycling talents. I was already a proficient runner, so I thought I could finish strongly in the last leg of the triathlon. As for swimming, I was definitely rusty, but I was comfortable in the water and had the mix of height and big hands that makes for speedy swim times. Triathlons were longer races, playing into my preference for endurance events. I now had motivation, but also opportunity: it was summer in Florida, low season for running races, and the relative cool of riding and swimming were appealing alternatives to broiling myself alive on daily runs.

After weighing out these considerations, I decided to look into doing a race. The initial question was exactly what kind of triathlon to sign up for. Just like running races, triathlons span a broad range of distances. I discovered that there are four main race distances, ranging from short races that take less than an hour to complete to massive Ironman triathlons, in which competitors swim 2.4 miles, bike a massive 112 miles, then run a full 26.2-mile marathon. *Had I read that right? 141 miles?* A race of that length seemed almost impossible. I decided to push myself, though not quite that far, and signed up for the Florida Challenge, a local triathlon located in nearby Clermont. It was an ambitious decision. The race was over 70 miles long, I was a novice in two of the three events, and the course featured a run longer than any I had attempted, even in a stand-alone race. I had only four months to prepare for this competition. My decision to go for it was a testament to my confidence in my abilities and approach—a hard-won self-assurance that had emerged as my body had shrunk. But whether this confidence was warranted remained to be seen.

# Drowning in My Own Talent

---

*Well, me don't swim too tough so me don't
go in the water too deep.*

—BOB MARLEY

There was no getting around it: the Florida Challenge opened with a
1.2-mile swim, so sooner or later I was going to have to dip a toe in an
actual body of water. While 1.2 miles seemed like an awfully long way
to go, I thought it would be manageable. I knew how to swim, I wasn't
afraid of the water, and, according to my parents, I had been the first kid
in my swim class to go in the deep end of the pool. As someone so naturally adept at the dog paddle, could I possibly struggle with swimming?

The campus pool was an outdoor Olympic-sized behemoth teeming with scantily clad swimmers of both sexes. I quickly saw that no
one was dog paddling. The lap swimmers were using mysterious hand-
paddles and kickboards as they moved effortlessly through the water. I
was a fish out of water and I hadn't even gotten in yet. I lacked goggles,
wore surfer shorts, and had failed the manscaping requirement of being totally shaved. I could handle looking out of place; I was, after all,
something of a pro at that game.

I found that I was no longer a natural in the water. Swimming experts
say each swimmer's stroke is unique, almost like a fingerprint. Mine re-

sembled a man simultaneously drowning and fighting off a shark attack. Different doesn't necessarily mean bad ... but sometimes it does. Where to even begin? My biggest problem was my inability to simultaneously swim and breathe. Most swimmers use a highly efficient freestyle technique, swimming with their face in the water and turning to either side to breathe. I attempted to emulate the strokes of those around me and managed a credible impression for a few seconds. After three or four strokes, I turned my head to the right, seeking air, but instead inhaled a copious amount of chlorinated water. Still in need of precious oxygen, I picked my head up out of the water to reacquaint myself with our planet's gaseous atmosphere. This was a bad idea, as it instigated a disastrous chain reaction: My legs sank like stones, with my hips in hot pursuit. Now as hydrodynamic as a boulder, my head bobbed under as well and I sucked in pool water yet again, resulting in further undignified splashing before I managed to regain the surface. Clearly, my habit of regular respiration was at odds with this sport.

As I resurfaced, I saw that a lifeguard was now standing over me, buoy in hand, looking concerned. She wasn't the only one. I struggled as casually as I could to the end of the pool and attempted to calculate whether I was (as my parents claimed) a "natural." Let's see ... it had taken me three minutes to cover fifty meters. The distance I'd have to swim in the race was 1.2 miles, which worked out to, umm ... about 2,000 meters, another thirty-nine lengths of the pool. At my current pace, that would take (more math, carry the three ... ) approximately two hours. As the cutoff time for the swimming leg of the Florida Challenge was only one hour and ten minutes, this could be a significant problem. Not to mention my current dilemma of getting back to where I'd started. With great effort, I quasi-swam across the pool without submerging (the lifeguard was now pacing along the side, making no pretense about the fact that she expected to effect a rescue at any moment). After only a single lap, my shoulders burned and I was out of breath. I had no swimming stamina, and things were only going to get more difficult from here. Having a lane to myself in a pool was a luxury I would not enjoy during actual competition. In an open-water swim, I would have the added challenges of swimming against waves, navigating the buoys on the course, and avoiding the loose elbows and flying feet of my fellow competitors. Needless to say, I was pretty discouraged.

I worked at it, though. I bought some goggles and a more appropriate swimsuit (shaving my body was a concession I was not yet prepared to make). More importantly, I swam three or four times a week. Each visit brought an incremental improvement, and soon the lifeguards didn't look worried when I signed in to swim. I was still far, far away from attaining the effortless form of those populating the fast lanes at the pool, but it was clear that, with good weather and a little luck, I wasn't going to drown during the race.

# The Triathlon

*Never drop out, because if you finish your
legs will hurt for a week...but if you drop out
your head will hurt for months.*

—THOMAS HELLRIEGEL

As summer bloomed and then faded, my preparations for the race accelerated. New skills had to be mastered and old skills enhanced. In-water navigation, bike handling, and quick transitions between the legs of the race were all things I had to learn how to do. Triathlon was pretty damn complicated, far more than running ever was. The rules for a running race were simple: put on your shoes and follow the pack to the finish. While preparing for my triathlon, I was frequently paralyzed by decisions as seemingly simple as what kind of shirt to wear during competition. After you get out of the water, you're going to be riding a bike, so do you swim in your bike jersey, or do you swim shirtless? How do you even get the shirt on if you're wet? Do you towel off? I was lost, and I hadn't even gotten to the question of putting on pants.

Proper nutrition during the race was another issue. Completing the race would demand upward of 5,000 calories (to put that in perspective, that's almost ten Big Macs). The human body can only store a fraction of that in ready energy. In order to keep moving during a triathlon, it is imperative to consume food and drink on the course to replace the calories you burn. To me, eating for purely utilitarian reasons was an entirely foreign concept. There are differences between this type of eating and the kind you do every day. During exercise, the taste of food becomes subordinate to how well your body digests it while in motion. Triathlon was expanding my horizons, and forcing me to adapt, learn, and expand my capabilities.

Since I lacked an experienced mentor to guide my progress, the task of designing workouts fell to me. The race in its entirety was far too long to duplicate in practice, so I devised ways to simulate pieces of it. For example, I would go to the pool in the morning, swim a number of laps, then tear out of the pool and run to my waiting bike, where I would immediately change and ride a few miles. My sudden, frantic exits from the pool frequently raised a few eyebrows; it must have appeared as though I was trying to escape from the swim practice in the adjacent lanes. Each time I pedaled away I had to bite my tongue to avoid yelling, "So long, suckers!"

Moving directly from swimming to biking produced an interesting sensation. While I was swimming, blood moved into the top half of my body, and I felt a little dizzy and weak in the legs after shifting from a horizontal position to the more upright pose of a cyclist. But while it took a little time to get completely comfortable, the swim-to-bike transition was a piece of cake compared to the bike-to-run transition.

To simulate the transition from cycling to running, I had begun to attempt runs immediately following my bike rides. I'd read about these workouts on the internet, where they were referred to (among other, more colorful terms) as "bricks." Depending on who you asked, the term brick came from either (a) the feeling in your legs during the run or (b) a portmanteau of <u>B</u>ike + <u>R</u>un = <u>ICK</u>. Either way, the experience didn't sound like a lot of fun, but I was dubious as to whether the feeling would be as bad as the hype. Running was my strongest sport, and I would be careful not to destroy my legs on the bike, part of my plan to minimize the ickiness. My first attempt at the brick workout was a

30-mile ride followed by a 7-mile run, both distances I had easily covered separately. I finished the ride, parked the bike, changed shoes, and proceeded to run. It felt like I was wearing two left shoes. I tottered along, wondering if it was too late to get my money back from the race registration (it was) and whether it was possible to do the run using a wheelchair (it wasn't). Amazingly, after two miles of this, my legs began to function adequately, and I was able to run normally again.

I later discovered that the reason for the odd sensations was that, while biking, certain muscles in your legs and hips cease to expand and contract, and they shorten over time to accommodate the seated position and the pedal stroke of the cyclist. When the cyclist abruptly becomes a runner, the results can be comical. As with swimming, I eventually adapted to brick workouts, as my running muscles learned that they would be needed after I finished riding. Just to be on the safe side, I told them. "We're almost done biking! Get ready to run!" I would yell as I coasted to a stop. While all of this happened, I was shoring up a thousand other deficiencies simultaneously. At some point it dawned on me that I was about to attempt an over seventy-mile triathlon. Who would have guessed I'd ever try something like this?

My last training day before the triathlon offered one more bit of fun I hadn't yet had the pleasure of experiencing. In order to become as aerodynamic as possible, I decided it was time to shave my legs.[13] I barely recognized my legs after I was done: bizarrely smooth and totally at odds with the rest of me. Just to even things out, I decided to shave my arms ... then my chest ... and finally, my back. This last job proved a bit difficult: I couldn't reach everything with a razor. I had Nair, but needed some sort of implement to spread the goo across my back. After a lengthy search, all I could find was a kitchen spatula. I slathered the business end of the tool with depilatory cream, covered my back, tossed the spatula back in the kitchen sink, and headed for the shower. Ten minutes later, I was toweling myself off when I heard my roommate

Seth moving around in the kitchen. As I came out, I realized he was cooking something. It was a grilled cheese, and he was turning it using the spatula I had just used on my back. I checked the bottle to make sure Nair wasn't too toxic and kept my mouth shut.

My triathlon debut marked the first time I had traveled overnight to a race. I had recruited my friend Ben as a sherpa, to provide both vital moral support and even more vital physical support, as I anticipated being pretty exhausted after what would be the most demanding event of my athletic career. The day before the race we drove south from Gainesville to the race site in Clermont. I knew I was pushing the envelope by attempting this race, so I'd deliberately selected an "easy" course; Clermont was near Orlando, deep in the pancake-flat state of Florida, and I expected that the greatest elevation change in the racecourse would be a bridge. I received a rude lesson in geography as we entered Clermont. There were hills. Big hills. Rolling hills. Hills far larger than the little bumps I'd ridden in practice. Later, I learned that Clermont was the home of the U.S. National Triathlon Training Center, chosen for its rare combination of varied topography and year-round warm weather. I remembered my experiences with the hills at Gate River and felt my pulse go up. I had unwittingly signed up for one of the hardest races in the United States. "Little hilly," Ben said, making a solid play for understatement of the year. Adding to my worries, Florida was in the middle of an unseasonable fall heat wave, and the temperature was forecasted to push ninety degrees that day.

Later that afternoon at the event registration, I was given reams of forms to fill out, most of them absolving the race directors of responsibility for my death by a wide range of enumerated eventualities. I signed my life away and was issued a swim cap and a large number of stickers to attach to my bike and person (the triathlon equivalent of toe tags, I thought wryly). With few rights left to sign away, I wandered with Ben down to the swim start, and I got to see just how far 1.2 miles was outside of a pool. A long line of buoys stretched away from shore, seemingly to the horizon, eventually paralleling the shore before returning to the beach some distance away. "Can you swim that far?" Ben asked. Theoretically? Yes. I had swum that far before. Once. In a pool. Now I had no idea. Seeing the distance in its totality made the difference between pool and lake seem less than trivial. For one thing, I saw far less to cling to in the lake, if I were to grow fatigued.

"Ben?" I said.

"Yeah?"

"Tell the world my story if I don't make it."

Walking back to the car, we noticed there was a small display set up for last-minute shopping. There was no reason to stop; I had all my equipment in order, and had already purchased the nutritional supplements and supplies I'd planned on using. We stopped anyway. The next thing I knew, I'd done something no reasonably intelligent person does the day before a race: bought a new piece of gear to use in that race. I had been having last-minute doubts about what I should swim in. I had planned on wearing bike shorts, but I didn't want to stand out or look like a stupid rookie (notwithstanding the fact that I WAS a stupid rookie), so I purchased a new swimsuit. But not just any swimsuit: a teeny, tiny, red and black Speedo. I felt almost naked wearing it. But I figured it actually solved my problem of potential embarrassment; I assumed that Speedos would be in vogue among the racers—otherwise, why would they bother selling them at the event?

Race morning arrived after a night of tossing and fitful sleep. I was a bundle of nerves. After setting up my bike and race supplies, I went to the final table to finish my registration. I told the volunteers my name, and the next thing I knew, a guy was slapping a little band on my ankle, like a park ranger tagging a particularly interesting wildlife specimen. I learned that this little ankle collar contained a chip that would register with timing mats around the course. "So you don't cut any corners," the volunteer said, attaching the band firmly around my ankle. I had other concerns: the neoprene strap appeared to contain quite a bit of gadgetry. "Will this shock me if I slow down?" I asked. The volunteer smiled at my joke. I was serious.

Now that I was safely catalogued, all that was left to do was mill around on the beach until it was finally time to go. I stripped off my civilian clothes and bared my Speedo, waiting for everyone to follow suit so I would feel less ridiculous. *Any second, everyone else will look just like me.…*

No. Of course not.

*Shit.* I was now standing in a Speedo, wearing the same kind of anklet someone under house arrest wears. Can you say "sexual predator"? Everyone else was wearing either bike shorts (only a few) or wetsuits (pretty much everyone). I got a few looks from people, as I stood out like a sore thumb. I pretended to be European as the countdown to the race began.

Other, better writers have described the start of a triathlon as a washing machine of flailing arms, feet, and elbows, which is as good a description as any. It's pure chaos, especially to a person new to both mass starts and open-water swimming. I fought for a tiny bit of open space to occupy peacefully, to no avail. Everyone was going so fast. Someone literally swam over me, and I began to hyperventilate. After an eternity (probably only ten minutes or so), the pack spread out a bit and I was finally able to find a rhythm and do some real swimming. As I took stock, I realized that the only reason I was alone was because I'd drifted off to the right, away from the direction of the swim course. I countersteered, making frequent corrections to my haphazard trajectory as I wove down the intended path of the swim course. Though I hadn't noticed it during the initial chaos, as the adrenaline wore off I discovered why people were wearing wetsuits: the water was rather cold, and I was experiencing severe shrinkage. This was particularly unfortunate given that my bathing suit left little to the imagination. I could already hear the one-liners upon my exit from the water.

After far too long, I reached the lonely orange buoy marking the turn-around point and headed back toward the now impossibly distant shore. Few thoughts crossed my consciousness during the swim. I wondered how I was doing. I had lost all sense of time. It was getting lonely out there. Unbidden, a thought from a dark corner of my mind suggested I might be in last place, with only a kayak or two behind me, ready to fish me out when I didn't make the cutoff time. In a flash, my insecurities took hold, and I was back at

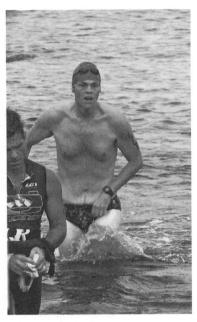

The infamous Speedo. Florida Challenge, Clermont, Florida.

my very first 5K race. I dared not look back, lest I see no one behind me. I was jarred from my self-pitying reverie when I literally jammed an arm into the soft bottom of the lake. I had reached the shore and the water was shallow enough to stand up in. I slogged ashore; 1.2 miles down, 69 to go.

It might be paranoia, but I think I heard a few chuckles at my (lack of) outfit. I jogged into transition number one feeling somewhat sea-sick. Swimming had left my legs without much blood and I was a little woozy. I imagined fainting and waking up in the ambulance to an EMT saying, "The Speedo's too tight. We'll have to cut it off." Clinging to consciousness, I struggled into a pair of bike shorts and a sleeveless jersey, grabbed a helmet, and was off. My stopwatch read a little over fifty minutes—slow by most standards, but by no means shameful.

The bike portion of the event was more familiar to me than the aquatic element, but still a relative unknown. In my dreams the night before, the foothills had spurted upward, turning into mountains before my eyes. I fell asleep saying a prayer that what we'd seen on the drive in wouldn't be representative of the terrain for the bike course, and the race would be flat, windless, and fast. No such luck. If anything, the course was hillier than I expected. The one good thing about being a slow swimmer is that I found plenty of slow cyclists to pass. With each person passed, I felt a thrill that drove me to hammer the pedals a little harder, a self-perpetuating motivation that had me moving up rapidly, albeit at the expense of a lot of energy. Depending on the terrain, a 56-mile bike ride is a two-and-a-half- to four-hour affair for most human beings. Sensitive to the length of the race, I backed off a bit, hoping to save my legs for crunch time. I finished the bike portion in a smidge over three hours; I was now doing quite respectably in my first triathlon. The last leg was my strength, and I was about two hours from completing a solid debut.

There are the plans you make, and then there's what actually happens. This was one of the times when they didn't match up. The wheels fell off. Things went to hell in a handbasket. Pick your cliché; the point is, I physically fell apart on the run.

This may have been unavoidable. Make no mistake; I'd been training hard, perhaps beyond my capacity. The wear and tear of training on my body had manifested in the form of some nagging injuries I developed weeks before the race. In particular, I'd been having an unusual problem in the muscles deep in my hip and buttocks. A deep, aching pain would emerge from nowhere and would severely curtail my range of motion, making it literally impossible to run. Rest from running alleviated the problem, but I was worried about losing fitness and had trained through it. During the biking portion of the race, I felt a few twinges in my leg but had soldiered through, hoping that they would go away.

On top of this, the weather wasn't cooperating. The race was scheduled to go off at 7 AM, allowing the athletes to take advantage of the cooler morning temperatures, but a delay of nearly an hour meant the day was already a broiler before we'd even begun. While we waited to start, the race DJ decided to spin the Nelly song "Hot in Herre," an appropriate choice, as I could feel the mercury rising while I stood on the beach. By the time I hit the second transition of the race, I'd spent more than four hours doing strenuous activity in high temperatures, and the three bottles of Gatorade I'd consumed during the bike segment were insufficient to replace the fluid I had left on the course that day. Together, all of these circumstances were proving pretty hard to handle, and I was hurting and just plain tired.

By themselves, none of my errors or misfortunes were necessarily critical. Their combined effect, however, was devastating. I'd made it through the transition zone and onto the run course, feeding off the energy of the spectators. As soon as I left that supportive cocoon, an unusual hollowed-out feeling hit me, starting in my stomach and working outward into my limbs. It was total exhaustion, and it felt like having a panic attack when you're already dead tired. My heart rate began to spiral out of control, and I was working exponentially harder to continue running at the same slow speed.

After a day full of mistakes, miscalculations, and blunders, I finally did something smart: I stopped at an aid station and took a walk break to consider my predicament. Like Scrabble tiles, I laid all the facts out in front of me. I had covered three miles and still had ten to go. My heart rate was coming down while I walked. My legs were still rubbery and I was so tired I was almost sleepy, at the edge of complete exhaustion. I arranged potential scenarios, trying to figure out the best way out of this jam. It was apparent that I had only bad options to choose from. I was probably going to have to run/walk the rest of the race, no way around that, but I was pretty good at managing my physical reserves, so I could minimize the time I would lose. I finished my walk break and started running again.

Only a few hundred meters down the road, things went from bad to worse to terrible. Without a whisper of warning, the cramping problem in my hip reasserted itself with a savageness that brooked no negotiation, only concession. I limped a few steps, tried to work the cramp out by punching myself in the hip a few times, and again tried to run. It was too much; fifty yards later I was doubled over, throwing up. Competing had never held a macho appeal for me, but I knew how to push my physical and mental boundaries. I also knew when my limitations were serious and when they weren't. This was serious. *So much for managing things.* I had only two options left: drop out and get a ride back to race headquarters, or walk the rest of the way to the finish line. There wasn't much to consider. I started walking.

Three hours and eleven minutes after beginning the run, I limped in, finishing close to dead last and feeling just plain dead. I staggered to the first piece of grass I could find and unceremoniously plopped down. I guess I didn't look good, because the finish-line volunteers visited me with paramedics in tow. So great was the categorical imperative to rest that I resisted the suggestion to go to the medical tent on the grounds that doing so would require me to get up.

After about thirty minutes of complete entropy, I was able to move under my own power. I shuffled to get my things together and headed out of town. Driving home that night, Ben looked over to the passenger seat, where I sat crumpled, staring out the windshield with a glassy thousand-yard stare. "Long day?" he asked.

"Long day," I agreed.

# Failure

*Our greatest glory is not in never falling,*
*but in rising every time we fall.*

—CONFUCIUS

When circumstance swats you down like an errant fly, you're basically forced to confront your failure. How you deal with it usually has more bearing on your long-term prognosis than how you deal with success does. I've mentioned that the obese are adept at rationalizing away their failures. To some extent, all people engage in this behavior. At one time or another, almost everyone has avoided facing up to the harsh reality that they just didn't get things done in the clutch. After all, what do you do when you've tried your best and still fail?

Having relied on trial and error extensively in my diet (and now in my athletic development), I was becoming something of an expert on handling negative results and dead ends. The worst thing to do in the wake of failure is to attach emotion or self-worth to the results. Nothing good ever comes from this. Since the first primitive human sparked fire, mankind has grown adept at deflecting and shifting blame to ignore our shortcomings. And if there's no one else to blame, people usually favor one of two coping strategies in the wake of a setback, both of them stemming from knee-jerk emotional reactions. The first strategy is to resort to banal platitudes: *You're a winner just for trying.* Such feel-good messages are counterbalanced by the second, even more hardheaded strategy for coping with defeat—to simply not acknowledge it. In failing to recognize failure, people who use this strategy maintain that anyone can achieve anything if they believe in it enough. Neither of these strategies seems to contribute to long-term success. While positive messages can salve your hurting pride, save your dignity, and make you feel better, these well-intentioned sentiments have one very dangerous side effect: they make it easy to feel justified in abandoning your goal too early or too easily.

On the other side of the coin, those who claim you should *never* quit under any circumstances are equally delusional. Let's be honest: there are things in life you are not capable of accomplishing, no matter how much you want them. History is peppered with examples of disasters arising from unrealistic expectations. Even if a goal is obtainable, you must weigh how desirable it is against the investment it requires. There are times when quitting makes sense, especially if the risks outweigh the rewards.

In reality, the truth usually lies between these two opposing emotional positions. A balanced consideration of your feelings, coupled with an objective assessment of the situation, will often give you a good idea of how to continue. However, for reasons that are not entirely clear to me, society seems to frown on frank self-evaluation. As George Bernard Shaw put it, "The power of accurate observation is commonly called cynicism by those who have not got it."

How you respond to your feelings in the wake of failure usually has more influence in determining your long-term success than the feelings themselves. It is implicit that most people attach a pejorative meaning to failure; they label failing as a negative, and usually want nothing to do with an activity they're not successful at. This attitude is OK if you plan on doing only things you're good at, but it's otherwise illogical. After all, failure is as common as success, if not more so. People typically go through several relationships before finding someone to marry. Is the salutatorian of Harvard condemned to a life of toil and drudgery for failing to be the best student? And, in the more immediate sense, had I and everyone else who failed to meet their goal for the triathlon (whether it was winning, getting a certain time, or even finishing) been a disappointment? The point: failure is rarely a clear-cut matter.

You often realize how much of yourself you're willing to invest in your goals in the wake of failure. After the triathlon, it was starting to dawn on me that my goals had shifted to the point where nothing was guaranteed. Coming up short was now a very real possibility; difficult as it was to accept, something as long and strenuous as a triathlon might be beyond me. After thinking about it, I decided I was all right with that. I came to realize that it was the very difficulty of the race that appealed to me; I craved the challenge, and if it had turned out not to be hard, I'd want to find something else that was. I was the only person I knew who had gone from being morbidly obese to being fit enough to even try something like this. I didn't know how much damage years of living at a high weight had done to my muscles and joints, but I was still determined to find out just how far and how fast I was capable of going. As I saw it, a meltdown here and there was part of the game; something's got to give. Either I'd push through and set a new limit, or, well…I'd walk the last ten miles. I wasn't afraid of walking anywhere. I signed up for another triathlon later that week.

The race experience hadn't been exclusively negative. While my physical performance had been far from ideal, I was pleased with the mental tenacity I had exhibited on the course. I had driven my body to its absolute limit and was proud to have done so. My failure, as I saw it, was merely the result of my ambition smashing into my current physical boundaries. How many people even give themselves the opportunity to discover if they can push that hard? I was also pleased with other aspects of my performance. I was happy about the fact that, even though

I was hampered by an injury, I was able to think clearly on the course to deal with my fatigue. Finally, I might not have gone fast, but I did finish the race, without even a thought of quitting. *That* was the result of months of discipline as well as pride won through the hard work of dieting and getting in shape. I had no doubt that, unless I was medically unable, I would in the future finish every race I entered or be pulled off the course in the attempt.

I probably *would* be pulled off in my next attempt unless I got my hip fixed. This was my first sports-specific injury, and it was inexorably chipping away at my athletic lifestyle. I could run only about two miles before it reliably flared up, at which point I was reduced to a miserable hobble. My biking and swimming were unaffected, but I had no illusions about my prospects for success in races while I was running a maximum of two miles in practice. This frustrated me endlessly. I felt as though I could spin my wheels as hard as I liked but would never make any meaningful progress. Most concerning, I didn't know what was physically wrong. I'd become increasingly concerned that what I was going through was in some way caused by wear and tear from being overweight for so long. If this was the case, I had bigger issues than competing in races: I worried about the prospect of a serious medical problem and how I would control my weight if I wasn't able to remain active. Put succinctly, the pain in my hip was also causing me some headaches.

One day at the lab, a number of us grad students were working to prepare scientific posters for an upcoming neurobiology conference. My friend Sean and I finished designing our presentations and headed over to the medical center's in-house printing facility to have them fabricated. We dropped off the graphic files with Roger, the facility's art director, and paused to chat about a few final instructions. During our conversation I noticed an unusual object in Roger's office. It was either a recliner or a torture device. I inquired, and learned that it was both: a massage chair. The story unfolded. Roger was a certified massage therapist planning to start his own practice upon retiring from the University of Florida. Since Roger was also a runner, I asked him if he knew what might be giving me problems, describing my symptoms in as much detail as I could in mixed company. Roger seemed reasonably confident that a little-known muscle called the piriformis was the culprit, and he asked if I'd like to have him take a peek and see whether this was the case. The term "take a peek" gave me pause. The piriformis is buried deep in the buttocks, so I had no idea what he had in mind. It was the middle of the day, and we were hardly alone in the middle of a busy printing facility. Normally, I would have taken a pass, but my hip was so painful that I was willing to do literally anything to gain relief, including opening myself up to an unprofessional molestation in the presence of a third party.

Roger led me and Sean into another room (darkened, I noticed with increasing anxiety), and asked me to lie face-down on the table they used for cutting posters. As I moved to get onto the table, Sean caught my eye and made a subtle nod toward the door, asking *You two wanna be alone?* I furiously shook my head, wanting some backup (or a witness in court) in case anything bad went down. Roger poked and prodded my lower back and the outside of my leg, and then, without warning, applied intense pressure to the outside of my right glute. For a moment, I was sure he had stabbed me. I screamed like a little girl getting a shot at the doctor's, and made a significant, if unplanned, contribution to the field of profane terminology. "That's the spot, huh?" Roger said, apparently unimpressed with his own ability to easily pinpoint the source of my protracted frustrations.

It *was* the spot. After work I went out for an easy run. After a single adjustment, I was able to run four miles with no pain for the first time in weeks. That night, I made an appointment to come by Roger's clinic later that week for a full working-over.

If the prospect of a sports massage excites you, you've likely never had one. It's like getting beaten up. In addition to the trouble with my piriformis, my quads and shins were a wreck from too much training. I spent a lot of time yowling and pleading with Roger to go easier on me. Over and over, Roger responded to my histrionics by calmly informing me that I needed a lot of work. No doubt about that; he squeezed so much fluid out of my overtightened muscles that my face swelled and my nose began to run while I was on the table. I was glad when it was over, and ecstatic the next day when I ran again without pain. After that first massage, I never suffered from piriformis syndrome again—I was back in business. Magic, thy name is massage. I became a repeat client, usually going in for treatment when I was doing a lot of training or when I felt soreness from overuse coming on. Roger was a very intelligent guy and a true professional, and he even gave me a discount (an especially welcome break for a poor student) in exchange for bringing him up to speed on the newest developments in neurophysiology. I'm eternally grateful I discovered the usefulness of a good massage therapist; if not for Roger, I might be a power-walker right now.

# Setting New Goals

*Continuous effort—not strength or*
*intelligence—is the key to unlocking*
*our potential.*

—LIANE CORDES

*Nothing is particularly hard if you divide it*
*into small jobs.*

—HENRY FORD

After the Florida Challenge, my 2005 racing season began to wind down. Almost everyone who participates in endurance sports needs an off-season to let the body recover and rebuild. There's a scientific principle, called Wolff's Law, that posits that any biological system, when subjected to a particular stress, will adapt itself to best handle that stress. Thus, it was unsurprising that I was getting faster as my body responded to the sport-specific training I engaged in. An extended break from competition provided my body time to adapt further (by growing new blood vessels, increasing the amount of oxygen I could take in, and adding different, stronger muscle fibers). Now that I was feeling healthy again, it seemed counterintuitive to take a break. Cutting back exercise to a basic level results in a loss in fitness in the immediate sense. In the long run, however, I hoped the break would allow me to reap a larger overall dividend upon resumption of regular training. In effect,

I accepted a short-term hardship in order to achieve something more important in the long term. Sound familiar?

I was in need of an extremely restful off-season, as I was planning a challenging year in 2006. I intended to begin my preparations to break through to the top distances in endurance competition after the New Year. For 2007, I planned to celebrate the five-year-anniversary of my fat-to-fit experiment by completing a monster-sized Ironman triathlon. This meant I had only eighteen months to get myself ready for the toughest mainstream endurance event in the world. It was a tall order, especially given the fact that I was currently struggling to complete races only half that distance. Preparing myself for an Ironman would not get done overnight. Like everything else I had done to lose weight and get in shape, it would be a process, one with many steps.

The Ironman triathlon is generally regarded as one of the longest and most difficult races in the world. First begun in 1978 in Hawaii as a test of who was the most fit—swimmers, cyclists, or runners—the Ironman had only a cult following until ABC televised the 1982 competition. During the event, cameras captured one of the most enduring images in sports: Julie Moss, a student competing to collect data for her master's thesis in exercise physiology, found herself as the surprise leader in the closing miles of the marathon. Pushed to the point of total exhaustion, Moss collapsed short of the finish line and crawled the final meters of the race. This image of perseverance captured America's imagination, and the popularity of the Ironman exploded. Over the years, Julie Moss wasn't the only person brought to their knees by attempting to cover massive distances at high speed. Each race consisted of a 2.4-mile swim, a 112-mile bike ride, and a 26.2-mile marathon, all done back-to-back with no breaks. Elite athletes take between eight and ten hours to finish, and amateurs commonly take the full seventeen hours that are allowed before the midnight deadline. Training is no guarantee of success; about 10 percent of the highly trained athletes who start any given Ironman will not finish because of heatstroke, injury, or overwhelming fatigue.

I had seen the Hawaii Ironman in person once before, as a child, on a family trip to Hawaii. I distinctly remember seeing the athletes prepare for the opening swim. The sun rising over the bay, sparkling off the clear water, and the hundreds of people with superhuman physiques and brightly colored swim caps made a powerful impression that lingered in the back of my mind for many years. I had seen the race in 1987, the same year I had begun to gain weight. Competing in this race myself, twenty years later, would perfectly symbolize that my physical health had come full circle.

I was hardly alone in my desire to complete an Ironman. In our bigger-is-better culture, people are drawn to attempt larger and greater feats just for the status they confer. The Ironman triathlon has become the "new marathon," and first-time competitors flock to races with little or no experience. Not all of these newcomers are willing to adequately prepare to fulfill their speculations or daydreams about the race. This rashness is often punished severely on race day. With an overall length five times greater than a marathon, each Ironman race sends many an ill-prepared competitor to the hospital.

I vowed to do whatever it took to maximize my chances of success. To initiate the process, I simply took out a piece of paper and wrote down the objectives I thought I would need to accomplish in preparation for this type of race. Here's what I came up with:

1. Run at least one marathon.
2. Finish at least one half-Ironman strongly.
3. Cycle at least 112 miles continuously.
4. Swim 2.4 miles in one session.

I planned my schedule around these goals. I had already signed up for a half-Ironman in May, which I hoped would take care of goal number 2. In the meantime, I would focus on completing each of the other tasks throughout the year. I began by signing up for the upcoming ING Miami Marathon.

A marathon was hardly a mere stepping-stone in pursuit of a larger goal. To this point, I had only run one local half-marathon and was still woefully inexperienced. And yet, as arrogant as it may sound, I thought running a marathon wouldn't be too difficult. This may have been out of mental necessity; the marathon was only one of three parts of the Ironman I aspired to. It would *have* to be manageable or I would have to question whether my goal was simply an overinflated ego trip.

To avoid another collision between my ambition and my limits, I trained diligently, following my training program to the letter. Marathon training is the same as preparations for any longer race, with a single long run each weekend. These runs start off at six miles and gradually built to twenty or more miles a few weeks before the marathon. After a couple of weeks of relative rest to rebuild your leg strength, you're (theoretically) ready to run a full 26.2 miles on race day. In late December I ran the Jacksonville Half-Marathon as a tune-up race, noting with satisfaction that I was getting significantly faster. Each Sunday, even over the holidays, I trained alone, grinding out the miles, rain or shine. I even bought an iPod to stave off boredom during the long runs.

My painstaking preparations were effectively washed away by a combination of imprudent action and plain bad luck. In the supposed "rest week" prior to the race, I was beset by the bane of the amateur athlete: work. I was up against a looming deadline and so was toiling around the clock in the lab when I was supposed to be relaxing. After a series of long nights, I made the five-hour drive to Miami the day before the race, arriving both stiff and poorly rested. As a graduate student living near the poverty line, I had opted for the cheapest accommodation I could find in Miami proper. "Cheapest available" turned out to be the South Beach Hostel, a noisy, crowded place full of waterbugs and people far more interested in partying than in recuperative slumber. I was assigned a small, stiflingly hot room with three Dutch students on holiday, hardly the makings of a good night's sleep. On the plus side, it cost twenty-nine dollars a night and was only a couple of miles from the race start.

That night, I met Jen, who had driven up from the Florida Keys to have dinner with me and provide a familiar face to help me stay relaxed and loose for race day. This touching gesture completely backfired. After saying goodnight, I was safely tucked in and drowsing when my ringing phone woke me. Jen was in tears; her car had been towed, and there was no choice but to come to her aid. We spent the next hour and a half reclaiming her car and searching for more change to feed my own parking meter. I wound up in bed again at 2:00 AM, worrying more about parking spaces than about race paces. I had slept fitfully and too little when my alarm sounded at 5:30.

Have you ever shown up to class and realized you forgot to study for a test that was being given that day? Toeing the start line, I felt like an unprepared student watching the teacher hand out the exam. My legs didn't have the spring they normally did, and I felt tired (never a good sign when you're still 26 miles and 385 yards from where you want to go). There was no sense in crying about things; I could only trust in my training and try to leave the feelings of flatness at the start line. Lamentably, my premonitions were, on this day, quite accurate. I got off to a good start, running the early miles at the pace I had trained for. The first half of the course was by far the most scenic; the race wound its way over the MacArthur Causeway into South Beach, where still-drunk partygoers were emerging from the clubs to find hordes of runners streaming down the empty streets. From there, the race proceeded north before crossing the Tuttle Causeway to rejoin the mainland, then turned south again, toward the halfway point at American Airlines Arena. I was in serious trouble by the time I reached the turnoff for half-marathon participants, who I watched enviously as they peeled off for their finish. I had maintained my pace nicely but was now running on empty.

The fat was already in the fire, and all I could do was stay focused and keep going. *Relax. Breathe. Drink at the aid stations. Just run this next mile. Then another.* The second half of the race took us south in an out-and-back loop to Coral Gables before returning downtown. Despite receiving a $250 parking ticket the night before, Jen had returned to cheer me on, and she was waiting for me at a cheer station at mile 21. When I came by, she later told me, it looked like I had died and was then somehow reanimated. In a photo she took, my face wears a combination of a grimace of pain and a lunatic grin. I remember none of this. *One more mile.* I was getting dehydrated now. The Miami weather was unseasonably warm, and I was losing the battle to replace fluids lost to sweat. In a cruel irony, I had loaded the audiobook for Stephen King's "The Gunslinger" on my iPod. The book recounts one man's solitary trek across a vast desert, dying of thirst and in pursuit of an ill-defined goal. It was appropriate. I was a shambling wreck at that point.

My recollections of the last five miles are patchy. My body was starting to shut down. At some point, I started taking short walk breaks to rest my battered legs. As I got closer and closer to the finish, the walk breaks got longer and longer. *One more mile.* I began to have irrational thoughts. A year earlier I had run a four-mile race that turned out to be five miles long. What if I arrived at the finish and it wasn't there? I managed to run the last mile, and the finish line was exactly where they promised it would be. I ended the suffering in just under four hours. Jen had beaten me there and was waiting for me at the finish. She called my name from only a few feet away, but I was apparently not holding office hours any longer. With nowhere left to run, my body quickly wound down. I shuffled through the post-race area, found a spot of grass, and half fell, half lay down, wishing only that there was some way to lie

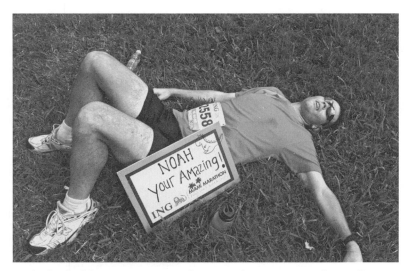

**At the finish of the ING Miami Marathon. Jennifer was too excited to spell correctly.**

down *more*. It was a full forty-five minutes before I felt I could even stand up again. My legs were totally destroyed, and I was massively dehydrated. Were I more coherent at that point, I might have considered the big picture and ended it all right there. *Okay, Mr. Big Shot, still want to do an Ironman? Think you can run this far after 114 miles of swimming and biking?* Fortunately, my brain was far too scattered for the thought to occur, although I was fully cognizant of the fact that marathons were pretty darn tough.

Jen was phenomenal after the race. Despite weighing only 112 pounds, she managed to lift and physically support me as we staggered the cruel half-mile to my car. Before the race, I had tried not to think about what four hours of continuous exercise would do to my body. As I peeled off my clothes, I had no choice but to see the damage. Underneath my crusty running attire, I was sporting a shocking array of wounds. In addition to the dehydration and exhaustion issues, I had some *really* spectacular bloody blisters; several toenails had already taken their leave; and both my nipples had been rubbed raw and had bled copiously down the front of my shirt. Despite these injuries (or perhaps because of them?) I was experiencing the strongest runner's high I've ever felt, and was so grateful to be alive that I somehow forgot that I had done all of this to myself.

After taking stock of the damage, I rejoined Jen to hang out for a little while before going back to Gainesville. From years of experience in a girlfriend capacity, Jen knew just what I needed to feel better: about five thousand calories. She rushed me down the beach to the Cheesecake Factory in Coral Gables. One of the best things about running a race is that you can eat almost anything you want immediately after. What followed nicely salved the pains of the race: fried macaroni and cheese balls, dinner salad, french bread and butter, a Portobello burger, and a piece of apple-pie cheesecake (and part of Jen's slice), all washed down with raspberry iced tea. By meal's end, I felt a little more human. I promised Jen that anytime she came to watch me race, we would go to the Cheesecake Factory afterwards for the caloric equivalent of a deadly sin.

On the way back to Miami proper, I noticed that the route looked a little familiar. "Wait a damn minute! I think I threw up in that bush about two hours ago. Didn't the race come through here this morning?" I squawked.

Jen had the good grace to look mildly embarrassed for selecting that particular route. I put a check next to "run a marathon" on my Ironman to-do list.

# The Rematch

*You yourself are your own obstacle—
rise above yourself.*

—HAFIZ

After a few days of stepping gingerly, I was back to doing a bit of training. In March I ran the Gate River Run yet again, navigating the course
in less than seventy minutes for the first time, thus setting another personal best. My attention turned to the pressing matter of the second
item on my Ironman preparation list, "Finish a half-Ironman strongly."
The event I had targeted for this purpose was the Ironman Florida 70.3
in Orlando. While the Florida 70.3 was the same distance as the Florida
Challenge I had completed in my first triathlon effort, the similarities
ended there. Though only twenty miles separate Clermont and Orlando, the terrain of each area is vastly different. Clermont is peppered
with steep hills, while Orlando is so flat that you can see the earth's
curvature. The Florida Challenge is an older, independent event that
built its reputation on being a tough venue for experienced competitors. In comparison, the Florida 70.3 event is a flashy circus, held in the
Disney Resort and run by the World Triathlon Corporation that is also
responsible for organizing the famous Ironman World Championships
in Kona, Hawaii. Four hundred athletes raced in Clermont, while over
two thousand would be lining up in Orlando.

Feeling cautious at the prospect of another total collapse, I was reluctant to invite a friend to witness my potential meltdown. So instead, I recruited my father to come visit and give me a hand at the race. He was the perfect choice for a wingman; he liked the spectacle of live sporting events, and as my father, he had already seen me both cry and crawl (two things I could not rule out from occurring during crunch time). Outside of the single race we had run together three years previously, Dad hadn't seen me race since I started getting in shape, and he was more than eager to come down and see what all the fuss was about. After driving down to Orlando (city motto: "Bring children and money") and checking into an iffy tourist-trap motel, we went to eat. In perpetuation of my legacy of questionable pre-race nutritional choices, I somehow arrived at the decision to consume a generous portion of calamari *fra diavolo* for my dinner. Food poisoning be damned; I feared no shellfish this week.

The next morning, I awoke to the same sound that had lulled me to sleep the previous evening: the explosive, yet somehow sonorous, noise of my father's snoring. It was the most annoying alarm clock ever. I suited up in an impressive array of brightly colored spandex, and we were off. Mindful of the fact I had suffered an energy bonk in my last triathlon, I kept a bagel in either hand as we drove to the race site.

7:30 AM on a cloudless May morning found me standing on the man-made beach of the lake in Fort Wilderness. I realized just how big-league this event was when I learned that the age-group waves of amateur athletes were scheduled to take off after the professional start. *Pros? Here?* I crowded to the front rank of spectators, eager for a peek at those who engaged in this sort of madness for a living. Seeing professional triathletes was a little underwhelming. The elite athletes looked like every other ripped person there. I found myself wondering what it was that made pros so special, but then remembered that I, of all people, should know not to judge a book by its cover. At the starting signal, the elite men took off as though it were they who had been shot from the cannon. Twenty-five minutes later, they had completed the swim and were on their bikes, and my wave was called to the starting line. I was racing as a Clydesdale (a competitor over 200 pounds), but was grouped to start with the 25- to 29-year-old men, a group chock-full of really fit studs. I myself was in good shape by any measure, but fifteen years of being flabby meant there was no way I would ever have six-pack abs. By now, I was using this sort of thing for motivation, and I was eager to see how many of the tri-studs at this race would be getting a good look at my back as I passed them.

We went into the water with the usual thrashing and aggressive maneuvering to establish good position for the rest of the swim. After a frenetic few hundred yards, I fell into a nice rhythm and began the serious business of swimming over a mile. My previous experience navigating in open water was paying off; I was able to sight off of the course buoys and swim in a much straighter line than before, which no doubt contributed to a speedier swim than the previous event's.

The Florida weather was, as usual, baking hot as I mounted my bike. We quickly left the confines of Fort Wilderness, and then the resort itself, as the course route took us on a tour of central Florida's finest back roads. I wondered why Walt Disney chose to build a resort in the hottest, most stifling part of Florida. I smelled some sort of conspiracy against me, but at least the course was flat, and I was very grateful for that. In addition to riding very conservatively, I was drinking everything I could get my hands on, as well as wolfing down energy bars and gels like they were going out of style. It's ironic to think that, after months of careful nutritional choices, I was now dumping fancy synthetic sugars into my body by the fistful, but I needed them to stay energized for when things would get tough.

Despite riding very much within my capabilities, I finished the bike segment faster than in my previous outing, in large part because of the lack of small mountains on the course. I started the run feeling, if not cool, then at least in control. My plan was to run the entire distance, stopping only at the aid stations every mile to refresh myself. I had gone about fifty yards when something truly bizarre happened: a little boy, perhaps three years old, ran out in front of me and yelled, "Hi Daddy!" while extending his arms in a plaintive gesture for me to pick him up. Thoughts of the race instantly evaporated as I scoured my memories of the past four to five years for an illicit rendezvous that might have led to the apparently illegitimate tyke now confronting me. No sooner had I pursed my lips to explain why he hadn't received a child-support check in a while then a woman I had never slept with scooped the little one up, admonishing him that I, in fact, was not his daddy. Feeling like a day-time talk-show participant who's just dodged a paternity suit, I veritably dashed away from my first brush with parenthood.

The run course comprised three identical laps, and two-thirds of the repeated path was on uneven grass or gravel. Whereas it had been merely hot on the bike, now it was boiling. I was chugging down liquids at every aid station and squeezing ice-water-soaked sponges over my head in a valiant effort to keep cool. People were wilting all around me, but today it was I who remained strong. After the first lap I spotted my father. "I'll be back in a minute!" I yelled as I made the turnaround. I kept my word, running the second lap strongly, but now even I was beginning to feel the combined effects of heat and fatigue. There was no witty remark for my father as I began the third and final lap.

All endurance athletes have unusual habits that manifest themselves in times of difficulty. Mine is to stick out my thumb when running, giving the appearance that I am either really enjoying myself (rarely the case) or subconsciously trying to thumb a ride to the finish (far more likely). Race photos from the third lap show me giving the rare double thumbs-up, a signal doctors might refer to as a contraindicator of my actual status. Aches were beginning to creep in, but they were the type

I could handle, certainly nothing catastrophic. I was on my way to my first strong finish in a long-distance triathlon. Five-and-a-half hours after plunging into the lake, I was approaching the finishing line, on pace to finish over a hundred minutes faster than in my initial attempt. As I neared the finish line, I saw the same kid who'd accosted me at the start of the run. "Who's yo' daddy?" I yelled at him. Amazingly, the tot grinned broadly and pointed at me. The gathered crowd, under the impression that I actually knew this child, applauded my acknowledgment of my (presumable) flesh and blood, and I finished to a stout (if undeserved) ovation.

In the finish area, the race organizers had set up a gigantic five-foot-tall misting fan. Overheated and cramping up, I was drawn to it like a bear to honey. As was true in the running world, I was a massive guy by the standards of triathlons and endurance sports. Too much mass and too few sweat glands rendered me unable to shed the high heat and humidity of the day as easily as shorter, smaller competitors. The only advantage my size conveyed was that now I was able to dominate the area in front of the fan for a full ten minutes, shamelessly using my bulk to block smaller athletes from edging in on my affair with the misty bliss it offered. I made a note to try competing in cooler temperatures. Still covered in sweat, Gatorade residue, and a hundred other terrible substances, I bear-hugged my father, ecstatic that he had been there for this breakthrough to the next level. I told him that he, as a good luck charm, was now compelled to come to my next important race.

Item number 2 on my to-do list: check.

# Robert's Tale

*You cannot wake a person pretending to be asleep.*

—NAVAJO PROVERB

Later the same day, my father and I had returned home and were sitting around talking with my roommate Seth, a fellow runner and soccer player. A little later, our third (and newest) roommate, Emily, came in. Emily and I shared a similar story, as she too had a history of weight problems. Driven by the goal of becoming fit enough to join a zoo management program in Gainesville, Emily had begun a program of diet and exercise. She was making wonderful progress, but had not yet returned to a normal weight. It was remarkable to witness someone else attempting something I knew firsthand to be so difficult. Naturally, I was supportive of her efforts, and I was very interested in picking her brain for thoughts on what it took to be successful. Frequently, we would compare notes and perspectives on the best approach to weight loss.

On this day, Emily was accompanied by her boyfriend Robert. They had been a couple for several months now, and it was an interesting match: while Emily was committed to getting in shape, Robert was going the other way. From what Emily told me, Robert had been steadily gaining weight since his high school track days, and, now in his late twenties, he was in the vicinity of 350 pounds, around what I had weighed at my peak. As he and Emily entered the room, the conversation turned to the race I'd just completed. Robert mentioned that he used to be a sprinter and somehow, after much posturing and propositioning, an impromptu footrace was arranged between him and Emily. A hundred-yard course was quickly set up. My father volunteered to be the official starter, and Seth and I split the timing and photographic documentation duties. Robert triumphed, but his 22-second time was almost twice that of a good high school runner. We strongly suspected that Emily had let him win to preserve his ego, and were preparing to voice our suspicions, when Robert doubled over and sat down. He was gasping, unable to catch his breath, and pounded on his chest and pointed toward his heart. In a nanosecond, the mood went from light to grim. Seth and I both had cell phones in hand, and I had punched in the first two digits of 911 when Robert finally began to regain his composure. After lying on the sidewalk for almost ten minutes, he managed to walk inside to lie down for a proper recovery.

It was alarming how the short race had affected Robert. In retrospect, we should have seen it coming. Robert's unrealistic outlook on his capabilities was evident from the statements he made during his frequent visits to our house. He appeared to feel pressure to rationalize his weight and would repeatedly mention that his size was a by-product of his job as a cook. He made the dubious claim that his boss "forced" him to eat entire portions of his dishes to ensure their palatability. As demonstrated, Robert also harbored wildly optimistic estimations of his own physical prowess. These were not limited to sprinting; several times, he mentioned that he considered himself a prime candidate for competing in mixed martial arts competitions. But clearly, he wasn't really in touch with what he could and couldn't do.

Watching the way our society treated Robert was a lesson in how the thin treat the obese. Robert had recently been diagnosed as pre-diabetic, and his restaurant faced the prospect of providing health insurance for an overweight individual who had now developed the additional comorbidity of a lifelong medical condition. Management, in all likelihood, found letting Robert go an attractive option. To avoid a discrimination lawsuit, they found a creative solution. Robert was transferred from basic food preparation to the job of pastry chef. Under doctor's orders to avoid sugar at all costs, Robert was unable to perform this new job, as he couldn't taste his creations to see if they were any good. As a result, he was fired. His next job was in the moldings department of a home-improvement store, but he was quickly injured in an accident and was placed on disability for some time. It wasn't clear if his injury was related to his physical condition, but Robert was certainly accumulating more than his fair share of aches and pains for a man not yet thirty years old.

Robert's behaviors (and the actions of others toward him) were typical of what I had observed of overweight people and served to confirm some of my initial suspicions about the culture of obesity. Particularly interesting was the interaction between Emily, an avid dieter and newly minted fitness enthusiast, and Robert, who was increasingly disinclined to live a healthy lifestyle. After they'd dated for a while, Emily recruited Robert to join her in losing weight. It was clear that Robert was madly in love with Emily and would do anything she asked of him, but while he liked the notion of losing weight, the practice of doing so was another thing entirely. This provided an interesting opportunity to observe firsthand what happens when a major change in lifestyle is attempted by a person who is not entirely committed. To his credit, Robert did lose weight in the beginning. He controlled his diet and exercised nightly with Emily. His body responded admirably to the changes, and he had visibly lost weight within a month. As if by magic, his pre-diabetic symptoms disappeared. I'd hoped that Robert would be motivated by these positive changes and subsequently galvanize himself to maintain a healthier state of being. Unfortunately, it became apparent that he wasn't going to make it that far. Cracks began to appear in the façade of his determination. Emily would catch him cheating on his diet during his lunch hour at work. She found pizza boxes in his apartment. He stopped going to the gym with her, claiming that he was (remember this one?) too busy. Slowly, almost imperceptibly, Robert slid back into his old ways. His weight loss slowed, stopped, and then reversed.

As his will crumbled, I noticed some changes in the way Robert spoke about weight loss. He would emphasize the healthy choices he made, but would rarely admit to making poor eating choices, even though Emily frequently caught him straying from the plan they'd agreed upon. In parallel, he began talking about the gym more than he actually went to it. As visits to the gym were more difficult to falsify than a covert Snickers bar, Robert would weave excuses: work was crazy, or his life was too hectic. In short, he was talking a bigger game than ever, but failing to back it up with his actions.

Emily was day to Robert's night. While he talked away his failures, she just kept working at her weight-loss program, quietly getting results. Emily was using rational thought to combat her problem, while Robert merely rationalized his. Rational thought (in the context of dieting) is an objective, critical evaluation of yourself, focusing on analyzing why and how you succeed and fail, with the ultimate intention of identifying a path to self-improvement. Rationalization (via manipulation of circumstance or perception) is designed to create an air of acceptability for failure to accomplish your goals. The former is useful not just for dieting, but for any major change in lifestyle; the latter is helpful only for creating a false sense of security in the face of adversity. Rational thought coupled with action is the key prescription for any successful lifestyle change. Rationalization coupled with inaction is a good recipe for falling back into the same rut.

Unsurprisingly, Robert eventually regained all the weight he had shed. It was clear that he had lost his own battle. But what about his relationship with Emily? What happens to a couple that diverges so widely on so basic a thing as physical maintenance? Would they grow apart or would they resolve this difference? As Robert assumed a more prominent role in Emily's life, she spent progressively less time at home and more nights at his apartment. With respect to her own weight-loss plans, moving in with Robert seemed about as useful as an alcoholic getting a job in a liquor store. Spending time with someone who's dedicated to rationalizing away the very problem you're struggling to overcome exposes you to validation for the thoughts that inevitably occur in your moments of personal weakness. Sad as it sounds, knowing that there is someone who will love you whether you succeed or fail takes a measure of wind out of your sails. At the same time, in an intimate relationship, each partner's health is so fundamentally intertwined with the other's that it's hard to negotiate major differences. As always seems to be the case, something (or someone) has to give. So what happened next with Emily and Robert was sadly predictable. By the time Emily had made the decision to officially move in with Robert, she had begun to gain her own weight back.

# An Unexpected Trip

*Be daring, be different, be impractical,
be anything that will assert integrity of
purpose and imaginative vision against
the play-it-safers, the creatures of the
commonplace, the slaves of the ordinary.*

—SIR CECIL BEATON

Having both run a marathon and finished strongly in my second attempt at a medium-length triathlon, I had accomplished two of the four goals I deemed necessary as preparation to compete in and finish an Ironman triathlon. This seemed like enough of a "deposit" to me, so I decided to actually register for my Ironman. Competing in the famous Ironman Hawaii was out of the question, as few spots were available to those not qualifying in another Ironman event. I investigated my other options, eventually settling on Ironman Arizona, held in April—twelve months away. IM Arizona was part of the wildly popular triathlon series that included the Florida 70.3, suggesting to me that the event would be well run (and wouldn't be arbitrarily canceled—losing out on a chance to race after investing a year and a half of training is the stuff lone gunmen are made of). The early spring date was attractive, and even if Arizona was baking hot by then, I would at least get to tell myself that "it's a dry heat." Before I could think better of it, I hit the "confirm" button, submitting my registration form. I was officially in; my rule for committing

to a race has always been that there's no going back once money changes hands. And with that, I was four hundred and fifty dollars lighter, so
I was already on my way to getting into race shape.

Now that I knew when and where I would be competing, the next
task was to coax a crew of helpers to join me. Judging from how debili-
tated I'd found myself after the comparatively short marathon, I knew
well that I was going to be in need of multiple caretakers after the Ironman. I made some calls, first to my father, and then to Jen. I figured
that, combined, they were strong enough to carry me to aid if I keeled
over. Both were incredibly supportive of what I was doing and bril-
liantly masked their probable distaste for spending their vacations in
the greater Tempe area. In particular, my father was very gung ho about
the whole idea. With his hip sidelining him from many sports, he was
excited that another Walton had taken up the cause.

There were many other things that needed to be done in preparation. Up next on my agenda was completing an Ironman-length swim
of 2.4 miles. While physically the easiest of the challenges on my slate,
this was still going to suck pretty hard. I preferred open-water swims for
my longer outings. For me, the idea that I am traveling from one point
to another alleviates the monotony of repeating the same motion over
and over. Florida's mild climate and plentiful lakes would easily accommodate this preference, if it weren't for the fact that alligators populate
almost every inland body of water, presenting a major hazard to swimmers who value their lives. Although seeing the same plastic band-aid
on the pool floor eighty times during a workout was depressing, I val-
ued my life enough to do the majority of my training in a pool.

I've never understood how avid swimmers don't go batty. The longest pools are only fifty meters long, and a good swimmer will swim
that distance several hundred times during practice, each and every
day. Looking at the same lane line continuously for even half that long
would give me repetitive stress disorder. Swimming could also be phys-

ically painful; goggles often ratcheted themselves into my head, growing tighter with every lap. When I removed them afterward, I would
have a clear impression of them around my eyes. Over the summer, my
back would tan and my front would remain a pasty shade of white, so
that my body resembled an unevenly cooked pancake. Nor was I terribly motivated to train at swimming: it was by far the least grueling
and shortest of the three segments in the Ironman. I made a deal with
myself: I would buckle down and commit to doing the basics to safely
survive the Ironman swim, but nothing more.

And then one day, I made a snap decision to forgo running and biking and just get the 2.4-mile swim over and done with. It stretched into
forever. The biggest challenge was counting laps (76 for the indoor
pool I was using), which can be quite difficult when you're getting dizzy
from going back and forth for so long. But finally, it was over. Getting
out of the pool was more of a challenge than the actual swim. Being
horizontal for well over an hour drew the majority of my blood supply
into my arms and shoulders, giving me Gumby legs as I struggled out
of the pool. I made a note not to try anything heroic on the bike for the
first few minutes during the actual race.

With goal number three safely in the bank, a single task remained:
a 112-mile bike ride to practice the distance I would cover during an
actual race. Biking accounts for the majority of the time and distance
covered in an Ironman. It was critical that I develop the stamina not
only to stay in the saddle for the six or more hours it would take me
to finish the bike portion of the race, but to have the legs to follow it
up with a marathon. I was not entirely unfamiliar with long-distance
cycling, having done several rides of around sixty miles in training for
other races. My longest outing had taken place the previous year, a 100-
mile "century" ride organized by the Gainesville Cycling Club. For that,
I had ridden within a group and was able to largely escape the drag of

wind resistance by riding in the slipstream of other cyclists, a tactic prohibited in triathlons.

As fate would have it, my work and personal lives intersected to provide me a unique opportunity to put in some time on my cycling. After toiling in the mines of graduate school for almost four years, I had made good headway toward receiving my degree. My progress may have been too good, in fact. I had been studying the function of neural stem cells and had performed a series of experiments that would demonstrate the usefulness of adult stem cells for certain therapies (my tenure in graduate school occurred at the peak of George W. Bush's "other war" on embryonic stem cells). Fortune had smiled on me, and I had already finished the research plan I had been tasked with by my supervisory committee. Having completed my course of study, I was looking forward to an early graduation. This sentiment was not shared by my research mentor, who viewed my impending departure simply as the loss of a productive worker, something that should be delayed. Rather than offering me a position as a postdoctoral researcher, my mentor opted for a stonewalling tactic, demanding I perform increasingly elaborate additional experiments. Never shy to assert myself, I informed my mentor that I felt he was asking for too much. This type of disagreement is common between graduate students and their mentors, and usually segues into a negotiation process leading to compromise over what additional experiments will actually be performed. On this issue, however, my mentor proved intractable. I was equally inflexible, as the thought of continuing to toil in poverty held little appeal. We had reached an impasse.

Apart from capitulating to my mentor's demands (and setting a terrible precedent for subsequent negotiations), I could see only one option for breaking the deadlock: going on strike. The graduate-student strike is a little-used tactic very similar to that employed by teamsters and other union members. All of a sudden, my experiments began to fail without explanation and my effort level dropped precipitously. Like any type of work strike, this was undoubtedly a dangerous move. A normally productive graduate student who becomes nonproductive has little reason to be kept on the payroll, and will be met by one of two responses: dismissal by firing, or dismissal by graduation. Given my track record in the lab, I was gambling that I'd be granted the latter option once it became clear that I had thrown down the gauntlet.

How does all of this relate to training for an Ironman? It had been almost two years since I had taken more than a day off, and I was sorely in need of a vacation. Sadly, the life of a graduate student is far from glamorous, and the pay supports few creature comforts beyond large quantities of ramen noodles and the occasional trip to the movies. So a luxurious vacation was out of the question. I decided to do something a little unorthodox instead. I wanted to repay Jen's kindness in coming to my recent marathon by visiting her. This could double as a vacation, since Jen worked as a dolphin trainer at a marine mammal park deep in the Florida Keys. Rather than drive, I decided I would make the trip to the Keys, almost 700 miles away, exclusively by bike. It would break down to four or five training rides of 100+ miles each. On consecutive days. In the middle of the Florida summer. With limited experience in biking for more than a few hours at a time, and with no plan for getting back home once (if?) I reached my destination. It may be unsurprising that, despite my best efforts, I was unable to convince any friends to join me.

My lab-mates made no bones about the fact that they considered me and my idea crazy. On the day I planned on leaving, they took me out for what they called a "goodbye lunch." Earlier that day, they had gathered to openly gamble on a "dead pool," placing wagers on how and where I was going to die on the journey. The leading causes of death predicted were dehydration/dementia, overwhelming fatigue, or riding into a swamp. Some of the more exotic long-shot scenarios included death by hobo attack, a redneck uprising, and contraction of the West Nile virus. No one picked a motor vehicle fatality, which surprised me. Would I have lived to collect, I would have put down a five on the wager that one of Florida's many bad drivers would take me out.

I set out on a Monday afternoon. I had budgeted four or five days for the trip, figuring the actual time would depend on how I felt and what sorts of things happened to me. My plan was to cut across the peninsula from Gainesville, arriving at the Atlantic Ocean just south of Jacksonville, at which point I would make a right and wend my way south to the tiny hamlet of Marineland (2004 census population: 10). There I would stay with Pavlo, my friend who was a graduate student at the University of Florida's beachside marine research lab. This first leg of the trip was a short hop of ninety or so miles, little more than a warm-up for the real work of the journey. I left town riding a wave of nervous energy. I felt good, and, although I wasn't in a particular hurry, I was making good time as the miles rolled by.

I strongly recommend biking to anyone thinking about adopting some form of regular exercise. At the recreational level, it's a low-intensity effort that promotes the burning of stored fat (as opposed to high-intensity exercise like running, which burns the "ready energy" contained in your muscles). You can maintain the level of effort required to cycle for long periods, and there's not a lot of pressure on your legs and hips, which is perfect if you're not in the best shape to start with. You can always move on to other forms of exercise later, if you want; this is not necessarily the case if you start getting into shape by diving into a more intensive form of exercise that can wreak havoc on untrained joints.

Cycling offers other benefits beyond those to your health. You enter a unique plane of existence when you stop driving and start pedaling. Even if you're just biking around town, things start to happen to you that would never occur if you were tucked away in a car. Other bikers and runners exchange friendly waves with you. You learn to savor the taste of chilly fresh air first thing in the morning. You hear the same kid practicing an instrument in his living room each day on your commute home. At parties, you can regale other guests with interesting tales of what you've seen lying on the curb (my favorite: an inexplicably abandoned pan of brownies). And by biking, you're doing probably the only thing that will simultaneously improve the environment and make you look better in the nude. It's a wonderful new world of experience.

As I slipped away from Gainesville, the scenery got less and less familiar. The city gave way to suburbs and finally to the back roads of rural northern Florida. This part of the state was clearly not designed with the comfort of the bicyclist in mind. The roads were narrow, with no shoulder or separate bicycle lane, and small hills abounded, exponentially increasing the risk of my being flattened by a cresting automobile. The road I was on was also traveled by huge semi trucks, which seemed (by the frequency of their air-horn blasts) to find my presence on the road less than welcome. Believe me, I wanted me to be there even less than they did. My inner peace was gone; I was pedaling furiously to reach more hospitable lands. Forty miles later I arrived in Palatka, a small town that provided a welcome respite as I stopped to refill my water bottles and rest my trembling legs.

In packing for this trek, I'd had to balance my need for certain gear with my limited ability to carry cargo. I wore only a small backpack, which I'd tried to pack with everything I would need. I had brought all of the essential gear: spare tires, tubes, and bike tools, a set of "normal" clothes, a map of Florida, my wallet, and a cell phone. In addition, I had packed a few luxury items: my digital camera and a pad of paper (partly to document the trip, and partly to give potential searchers some clue as to my fate). I also carried two water bottles on my bike's frame and had packed a gigantic bag of homemade trail mix (with a heavy emphasis on sweet dried cranberries and M&Ms), both staples of any outdoor adventure. Thus far, the trail mix and my water bottles were getting a lot of use, as I discovered that covering this much ground was hard, thirsty work.

As afternoon gave way to evening, I could feel the composition of the land change beneath me, as though the earth was preparing itself to give way to the impending sea. Perhaps all humans are born with such a sense, a reminder of the inextricable linkage of water and life. Or perhaps it was just the whipping late-afternoon ocean breeze I was now pedaling into. Judging from the strength of the wind, I knew the ocean had to be getting close. My legs grudgingly went through their revolutions again and again, as I paid dearly for the earlier bursts of panicked energy I'd expended to get away from the hostile truckers. After grinding down a featureless asphalt road, I was spit out onto the famed A1A highway in St. Augustine, a mere dozen miles from my destination for the night. I rolled in shortly before sunset and found a soccer game in progress between members of the marine lab. Pavlo had spotted my arrival and jogged over to ask if I'd like to join the game. Having covered the second-longest distance I'd ever attempted on two wheels, all I was capable of at the moment was to topple off my bike and lie down in the grass. I had cycled for only half a day and covered barely 10 percent of the total distance for the trip. I couldn't imagine any way I was going to make it to the Keys.

After a few minutes of indulging in self-pity, I got up and walked across the street to the beach. I plunged into the cool ocean, still wearing my cycling clothes. I was doing everyone a favor; I stank to high heaven. I floated on the rolling tide, watching the sun go down over the Intracoastal Waterway, and began to feel a little more *joie de vivre*. Cycling fatigue is a funny kind of tired: you feel worn out for a time, but you can bounce back fairly quickly. In the Tour de France, cyclists expend more energy than a typical marathoner every day, day in and day out for nearly a month, while elite runners are physically devastated for weeks after running flat out for only a couple of hours. Bike fatigue is just as much mental as it is physical. When you're tired, your optimism seeps away, and what's left are doubt and uncertainty about your abilities. At that point, you have to dig deep to find whatever it takes to keep going. Great athletes talk about this moment with reverence, and for good reason. The decisions you make when you're not feeling your best tell you what you're made of.

I was already somewhat familiar, if not entirely comfortable, with these low periods. I had gone through them before, both in sports and in life in general, and I knew what was needed to get my butt back on the bike the next day. Contrary to the claims of the motivational speaking industry, saying the right thing to fire yourself up is something no one can teach. Self-motivation is far too individualistic to predict or dictate; what will work for one person won't move someone else at all. Life experiences are critical to learning what you respond to best. There's just no other way to find out how to get yourself back on your feet than to put yourself in a position where you're knocked off of them. Coming up gasping for breath in my first attempt to run and falling apart in my first triathlon were only a couple of prime examples of very difficult experiences that were now paying off.

In order to keep going in the face of utter hopelessness, you have to push some pretty strong buttons in your head. I knew from experience that I responded best to a mixture of self-intimidation and fear of failure. One of my signature mental traits is a major aversion to what I consider self-embarrassment. This entails a strong fear of failing publicly. Taking the bus home to Gainesville after only one day of biking would, to me, suggest that other people saw me as a real weakling who talked a big game but couldn't back it up. I have no idea how psychologically healthy this tactic is, but if I have to scare myself in order to accomplish my goals, so be it. I had also been through the experience of trying to do more than I was capable of. Deep down, I knew that if I hit a point on this bike trip where I simply couldn't go on, I would have the brains to pull myself off the road and hang it up, knowing that I'd done the very best I could. On that first night, I wasn't there yet, and I was still able to envision finishing the trip one step at a time. Tomorrow I would get back on my bike and start riding south, but in the here and now I was going to get out of the ocean, take a real shower, and have dinner with my friend before my growling stomach actually bit me.

The next morning was gorgeous. Scattered clouds and low temps were predicted to pave the way to a brutally hot day, but in the cool morning breezes, I couldn't think of a single place I'd rather be. The night before I had crashed in the student dormitories and slept like a baby (an inestimable benefit of regular exercise). After a quick breakfast, I was ready to go. Pavlo escorted me to the edge of town in his car, honked twice, and then left me alone again with my bike and my thoughts. Leaving Marineland marked the end of the official itinerary I had laid out for the trip. I had no real timetable or hotel reservations to keep. There was no way to predict how much ground I could cover, or even what route I would take. The quickest and most scenic way at the moment appeared to be the A1A, so I followed that.

That morning was the best I've ever spent on a bike. The breeze coming off the ocean was fresh, tangy, and (unlike the previous evening's wind) at my back. The road was smooth, free of traffic, and laid out with a generous shoulder upon which to ride. For most of the morning's ride, I was no more than a stone's throw away from the beach. Once, an osprey flew over my head with a fish still wriggling in its talons. I thought briefly of what I would have been doing in the laboratory—probably mixing small amounts of clear liquids in a painstakingly tedious experiment. Out here, I was free and without a care in the world.

After lunch, the road took me inland on a far less spectacular route. I rolled along, not really thinking of anything but how hot it was getting. Though the air flow makes it easier to withstand, heat takes a huge toll on the cyclist. When I stopped at midday, I noticed that a thick crust of salt had formed on my backpack. I was drinking about two liters of fluid every forty miles or so, a sure sign that the weather was heavily affecting me. Perhaps the heat was affecting my judgment, for it was at this point that I began to blunder into some odd happenings. Late in the afternoon, I was traveling south, down the length of one of the outlying chain islands, and had just recrossed the Intracoastal Waterway to enter an unnamed town on the mainland. At some point I must have taken a wrong turn, as I lost the main road. Trying to get back on track, I resorted to using the sun to plot a southerly course, hoping the street I was on would rendezvous with the main road sooner or later. But no major thoroughfare was to be found, and in my search for it I strayed into a neighborhood comprised entirely of 1950s-era trailers. This trailer park was massive, the largest I've ever encountered (this *means* something, coming from a North Carolinian), stretching as far as the eye could see. The residents didn't appear dangerous (most were retirees, it seemed) but my attempts to retrace my steps failed, and I succeeded only in getting more turned around. The street I was on became narrower, then turned into an unpaved dirt and grass track. I stopped to consult my map, puzzling as to how I was going to get myself out of this surrealistic jam.

Searching for a reference point, I spotted a pair of railroad tracks running along an embankment above me and was able to locate them on my map. It looked as though, if I followed the tracks south, they would intersect with a number of major roads. From there, I should be able to reorient myself easily. The other option was to admit that I was lost and ask directions, a possibility I categorically rejected as a card-carrying member of the male gender. Decision made, I took my bike and walked it up the embankment and onto the tracks. I gingerly plodded along atop the tracks, taking care to not bang my bike against the railroad ties. After a few hundred yards the tracks climbed further over the surrounding land, rising to perhaps twenty feet off the ground with a short trestle separating the tracks from the steep, rocky embankment. As I appreciated for the first time how exposed my position was, I heard the familiar high wail that could only signal a train in the distance, originating in the direction from which I had come. It was relatively far off, but I had no way to easily escape. Jumping and/or sliding down the embankment looked rather hazardous, definitely a last resort.

A few hundred yards ahead, I saw signs for a train crossing, presumably indicating an intersecting road. It was a race then, with the train rapidly eating into my head start. I was further handicapped by the fact that I was awkwardly wheeling my bike and wearing footwear not designed for contact with the ground. Unlike regular shoes with supple rubber soles, bike shoes have a sole made from unyielding carbon or plastic, with a clip under the ball of the foot that allows them to connect to the pedal. I scampered down the tracks with an ungainly prancing gait as the telltale sounds of rolling stock drew closer and closer. The conductor spotted me and renewed the protracted blasts of the train's whistle. It was going to be close. Bare moments before being run over, I reached the road, where the embankment was shallow enough to allow me to jump off the tracks. As I tumbled away, I wondered who'd picked "flattened by train" in the lab's dead pool. Dusting myself off, I found I needn't have hurried to regain my footing; it was a freight train, easily a hundred or more cars long. Since it would be a while before I could get back on the tracks, I took a look at the road I had escaped to. Neither map nor eye told me that this was a main thoroughfare. Nevertheless, all roads lead somewhere, and it was worth venturing down a blind alley if it would get me out of this godforsaken town even a few seconds sooner.

The single lane of the road wound uphill for a few hundred yards, ending in a cul-de-sac containing a single dilapidated house that appeared abandoned. I turned my bike to execute a U-turn, but did so a bit too sharply and slipped. Preoccupied with staying upright, I was startled when a fierce-looking German shepherd broke cover perhaps thirty yards from me, charging me and barking like it meant business. To my credit, I kept a relatively cool head and grabbed for my water bottle to squirt the dog, hoping to thus scare it away. Naturally, my water bottle was empty, and the *pffft* it issued was insufficient to turn back the charging beast. Seconds away from a close encounter of the canine kind, I snapped. I was on an absurd trip, lost in a bizarre trailer metropolis, and, at the moment, I was a walking country music song: I was hot, tired, out of water, I stank, I'd almost been hit by a train, and people were wagering on how I was going to die. I would be damned if I was going down for something like a case of rabies. The dog wanted a piece of me? I wanted a piece of him. I charged the dog, screaming like a rabid zombie. The dog, realizing I was significantly larger and crazier than he, fled in the face of my countercharge. Ten minutes later I had found my road and was back on track.

The rest of the day proved less exciting, but by no means boring. The launch pads of Cape Canaveral gave way to strings of islands with long stretches of parks, occasionally broken by miles of planned developments. As daylight faded, the temperature dropped, and cycling became much more pleasant, almost to the point where I wished I could keep going. Almost. Around 6:30 I passed a small mom-and-pop hotel with a wistful glance, promising myself that I would stop at the very next decent-looking accommodations. An hour later, I was still pedaling along, having seen not a single place to stay. I was stuck in a suburban hell comprised of endless developments of cookie-cutter condominiums and vacation houses. These colonies, each of which proclaimed itself a seat for "luxury living," stretched mile after mile like a run-on sentence, unpunctuated by a gas station, supermarket, or anything resembling a room for the night. I had traveled almost two hundred miles since morning, and the sun had now slipped entirely beneath the horizon. The night air had cooled my sweaty body so that I shivered slightly with each breeze. I had exhausted my supply of trail mix several hours ago, and my water bottles had once again run dry. Although I was surrounded by people, I was getting worried—I was ill-equipped to safely ride at night and there was no telling how much farther shelter was. Five miles later, I nervously flagged down a policeman, who kindly informed me I was no more than a mile from the Vero Beach Hilton.

Walking up to the reception desk at the Hilton, I'm sure I looked like a real moron. For that matter, it's hard to muster very much dignity when trying to check in to even the seediest hotel while wearing spandex cycling shorts. If you ever find yourself in this predicament, I offer the following two tips: First, the "poor, tired biker" routine goes a long way in getting a discount. Second, if you're riding 100+ miles each day, you'll save a lot on expenses if you pick a place with a complimentary breakfast. Trust me.

The third day of my trip was largely uneventful. I had again slept well, and so, despite having covered two hundred miles on the previous day, I began the new day with fresh legs and rode fairly quickly. Once I hit my stride, I was capable of eating up some pretty big distances pretty quickly. This day's segment was somewhat shorter by design: I couldn't reach the Keys by nightfall, but I didn't want to stay in a pricey Miami hotel, so I traveled only as far south as Boca Raton (literal English translation: The Rat's Mouth). I made it there easily and stopped early to rest for the next day, which was going to be challenging.

The fourth day was indeed the hardest. After spending so much time in the sun and wind, my body was becoming severely weathered. My shoulders were sunburned and my lips had begun to crack and bleed. I was also getting saddle sores, which are almost less pleasant to describe than to experience. Once again, trust me.

I don't recommend traveling by bike through the Miami-Dade metropolitan area. Too much sprawl, bad roads, and even worse drivers make the route through Miami a nightmare for touring cyclists. Slowly, excruciatingly, I got through the worst of the city and resumed my southerly course. South of Miami, civilization began to dry up, appearing only in dribs and drabs on the various islands that constitute the Keys. Buildings became smaller, then farther apart, then nonexistent. The last landmark before the famous two-lane road that stretches all the way to Key West is Florida City, an ambitious name for three hotels and a handful of chain restaurants. Stopping briefly, I topped off my drinks and prepared myself to navigate the final thirty miles of swampy desolation. I called Jen and left a message regarding where she could expect to find my mangled, dehydrated corpse if I didn't show up in about two hours.

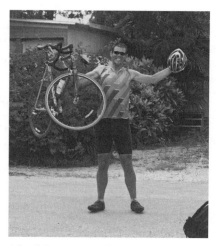

After biking across Florida, time to celebrate!

Thanks to the work of some forward-thinking soul at the Florida Department of Transportation, the road leading through the Everglades is lined with raised reflector strips, spaced every thirty feet for approximately fifteen miles. Though hardly noticeable to those traveling by car during the day these reflectors provide a continuous visual distraction to any cyclist navigating the shoulder of the road. I was dizzy and nauseated by the time I reached Key Largo, the first substantial island. I stopped across from where the eponymous movie was filmed and called Jen again to update her. I was pleasantly surprised to learn that it was only another five miles to her home, a mere trifle at this point. A few minutes later, I had made it. Jen rode her beach cruiser out to escort me in. It was the first company I'd had on the road all week.

Though I'd planned on returning to school immediately, I wound up spending two days in the Keys to recover. I was completely wiped out from my trip. Though it's not hard to sustain long periods of cycling over continuous days, once you stop for a day of rest, your body tends to rebel against any further activity. I was achy and stiff for the rest of my vacation, but I still had a lot of fun. Jen wielded her influence as a senior park official, and I was privileged to see all the critters, VIP-style. On Sunday, I rented a convertible, put the top down and my bike in the trunk, and drove back to where I'd started in about seven hours, fully appreciating the speed of the modern automobile. The next morning, I returned my rental car, and then, of course, I biked home.

In all, I had completed four lengthy bike rides, three of which were significantly longer than the bike segment of an Ironman. Overkill? Perhaps, but I could confidently check the goal off my list. I was pleased to find that I was officially ahead of the schedule I had set for myself, having accomplished all of my major training benchmarks with months to spare before the race. And there was another happy consequence of my long training jaunt. Though my co-workers were aware of my plans, no one had bothered to tell my mentor that I would be gone. A normal boss might have been angry or upset that one of his employees took time off without informing him, but my mine was a complicated fellow, driven by emotions and motivations few may understand completely. Upon hearing that I had abruptly left to bike across the state in the broiling month of July, my boss was less irritated than concerned about my apparent mental instability. When I returned, he called me into his office for a chat. It quickly became apparent that he viewed my actions as some sort of suicide attempt or cry for help. It seemed to me, though he didn't use quite these words, that he thought it likely I would do something like this again if left to my own devices, probably killing myself and making him the mentor who drove one of his students to commit suicide. Therefore, my mentor informed me, he had decided to reconsider his position on the status of my studies. I was given permission to begin writing my dissertation and to set a date to defend it. It was the beginning of the end of my time as a student.

# One Big Weekend

*As human beings, our greatness lies not so
much in being able to remake the world...
as in being able to remake ourselves.*

—MOHANDAS K. GHANDI

Rather than a gentle winding down, the months following the announcement of my graduation brought me more work than ever before. In addition to compiling four years of nonstop experiments into a presentable dissertation, I began the time-consuming task of identifying labs at which I could pursue postdoctoral work.

With the frenzy of activity that engulfed me, this was perhaps one of the only times in my life when I was legitimately too busy to be involved with anything athletic. In spite of the excitement associated with my impending life change, I became bored. Spending fine fall days hunched over a keyboard was quickly wearing thin. I had physically changed on such a basic level that I almost felt ill if I wasn't exerting myself toward a significant athletic goal, and my attention span was suffering as well. I was fresh and fit after my summer of training, and I found myself continually casting about for another race to do. On the spur of the moment, I found and selected the Miamiman triathlon, a quickly upcoming half-Ironman held adjacent to the Miami Metrozoo. The race held a certain allure for my competitive nature, as it served as a regional qualifier for the national triathlon championships run by United States of America Triathlon, the governing body for the sport of triathlon in our country. With this carrot to dangle, the Miamiman was sure to attract a quality field against which to test myself.

A wrench was thrown into my haphazardly laid plans a week later. I had been working on arranging a time to present and defend my dissertation, the last and most significant barrier to graduating. Getting the four busy scientists on my dissertation committee together was a lot like herding cats, and the only open date I could find was a scant two days after my race. With only thirty-six hours to reprogram myself from sportsman to scientist, pulling off the double feature would definitely be a challenge. But scratching myself from the race was out of the question, as the event had developed into a veritable social spectacle. My father was now coming down for both race and defense, and my roommate Seth and his girlfriend both were both in the mood for a trip to Miami. When Jen also agreed to attend, the race turned into a regular party.

The week of the race was spent in feverish preparation for my defense, and I was still short a few charts of data when my father rolled into town to collect me for the drive to Miami. I had no time to mentally prepare myself for the race; my life felt like it was happening in fast-forward. Later that night, our group rendezvoused in South Beach for dinner. The combination of the warm ocean breeze, an excellent restaurant, and good conversation conspired to draw dinner out, and it was well after midnight before we returned to the hotel, leaving me a grand total of four hours of sleep before the alarm would sound. To safeguard my rest, I had banished my father to his own room, where his snoring would not disturb me. I shared a room with Jen instead. While Jen is adept at the art of slumbering in silence, she failed to understand my need to show up on time for the race. When the alarm sounded, Jen turned it off and rolled over, apparently intending to go back to sleep. When I questioned this action, she suggested that we just keep hitting the snooze button because it was too early to get up. "I don't get out of bed for less than $9.25 an hour," were her exact words. I, however, did.

Grumbling something to this effect, I coaxed Jen out of bed and prepared to mark myself with my assigned race number. For most races, competitors have their numbers written on their arms and legs in permanent marker. As Jen stenciled the numbers onto my quads, I noticed something: My race number was 707. From my upside-down perspective, the numeric palindrome read "LOL."

Upon arriving at the race site, I found that Miamiman's swim was laid out in a double-loop course, with a complicated series of turns. As someone with only mediocre navigation skills, I was definitely not feeling ready to LOL about this. But despite the Byzantine layout of the course, I swam well, setting a new personal best that was no doubt aided by the wetsuit I had finally bought. The first transition zone involved a run of over a quarter-mile on rough pavement, which left my feet feeling as though I had just taken them across a pile of smoldering coals. The bike course was flat and troubled by only the slightest bit of wind, taking riders through some surprisingly rural parts of unincorporated Miami. The bike segment of a triathlon is often a crucial turning point that can have a huge effect on how the day plays out. One of the major questions you must decide on the bike is how fast you want to go. There's a delicate balance to strike: going too slowly means needlessly surrendering precious minutes, while going too fast toasts your legs before the run even begins. According to my bike computer, I was poking along at almost the same speed that I had gone earlier that year in the Florida 70.3 event. I wondered if I could ride faster. In the course of completing the goals I had set to prepare for the Ironman, I had trained harder and longer than I ever had in my life. I had confidence in my fitness, and I knew that probably the only thing holding me back from a breakthrough was located in the six inches between my ears. I had to be prepared to reap the rewards I had worked so hard to sow. I stepped up the pace.

My third try at a triathlon was indeed the charm. For the first time during a race, I was in the zone. I ate just the right amount of calories, drank the right amount of fluids, and exerted myself perfectly. Even after posting a personal-best time in the bike segment, I came back in ready to run. I would have felt even better if I'd known that my fast bike time had put me in contention to claim one of the coveted qualifying spots for the U.S. national championships.

I was racing in the Clydesdale division (the big men). The race offered qualifying spots for the national championships to the top three finishers in each division. After my slow swim, I'd been well off the pace, but thanks to my strong bike ride I had moved into fifth place in my division. In the opening mile of the run I passed another competitor to move into fourth and, while I didn't know it, I was only one place away from a qualifying spot. Conditions were warm, but the sky was overcast enough to make me feel comfortable in pushing the pace a bit. I was passing people easily, many of whom were incredulous to see such a big guy moving so quickly. Three miles in, I came up beside two guys who were running together. "Nice cadence," one of them said as I passed, in a tone suggesting that he thought I was pushing too hard in the early going. But that was the last time they saw me, as I passed them both. Midway through the first loop of the course, I saw Seth and his girlfriend, who had soldiered through the morning after a late night of partying to come out to support me during crunch time. I waved and pressed on.

Naturally, inevitably, I was beginning to feel the effects of the day's circumstances and my increased efforts by the end of the first running loop. My father and Jen were at the halfway point, yelling encouragement. Usually I hear everything while racing, but that day I was barely aware of what was going on around me. I was struggling to stay in the zone, thinking only of two things: I was having a great race, and there were still ten thousand meters between me and the finish. At the beginning of the day I'd thought there was zero chance of my getting a spot in the national championships. Sure, I'd been improving, but the competition here was too deep, wasn't it? Now, however, things weren't so cut and dried. Although I wasn't completely certain of where I stood, I was on track to qualify if I could keep catching people. Less than a mile later, I had my chance. A beast of a guy, definitely in my division, was struggling mightily in front of me as I turned a corner toward the zoo's main entrance. As we reentered the zoo for the last time, I made the pass and there was no response. A minute later, I chanced a glance back; I was still moving away and opening up a gap. Even though I was now in position to nab a qualifying spot, the only way to make certain of this was to keep pushing, lest someone behind me get a second wind. Rather than be caught myself, with less than two miles left, I caught up to another competitor with a "C" (the symbol for a Clydesdale competitor) on the back of his calf. This was the guy in second place. He was still running pretty quickly, and it took me several minutes to span the fifty yards separating us. I tried to ease by, but unlike the previous fellow, this man was ready to fight for his position. He fell in and matched my pace.

As we ran, stride for stride, I pondered what to do. Previous experience in running races had taught me that I was not blessed with the physical attributes of an elite athlete. My cardiovascular abilities were merely average, and I would be able to summon little speed should this come down to a final sprint. It was imperative that I drop this guy from my coattails before we neared the finish line. But how? I decided to employ an old trick. Just before the last aid station I eased my pace sharply, feigning fatigue (an effect requiring little exaggeration) and allowing my competitor to take the lead. As he slowed to grab water for himself, I skipped the aid station and hit the gas, gambling that I would catch him flat-footed and manage the last mile without cramping up from dehydration. It worked. With my competitor caught unaware, I opened up a lead and didn't look back. My world narrowed in focus as I squeezed everything I could from my tired legs. I reentered the park hosting the race. There were two hundred yards left. Then a hundred. Finally I crossed the line, ultimately taking second place and securing my spot in the U.S. national championships for the following year. Having pushed myself harder than I had ever dared before, I was accordingly depleted. I left the finish area and plopped down by an ambulance, just in case. That afternoon I made my first podium appearance at a major race. To celebrate, my supporters and I observed a burgeoning tradition to which I was quickly becoming accustomed: lunch at the Cheesecake Factory.

After eating, it was time to head back to Gainesville. Getting a dream finish was elating and draining in equal parts. On the way home I fell asleep like a baby, but one that was too large for his father to carry inside at the end of the drive. The next morning I was sore and tired, but my brain was energized and prepared for what I hoped would be the final presentation of my student career.

Some of the biggest effects of losing weight and adopting a healthy lifestyle were actually mental. Not only was I happier in general, my cognitive functions were clearer and more concise than ever before. I had started the process of weight loss at the tail end of my undergraduate career, and had lost the majority of my weight—over a hundred pounds—before beginning graduate school. The best way to characterize the cognitive shift is to say that it felt as though a pall had been lifted from my thought process, one I wasn't even aware of until it was gone. My mind was sharper. I could remember more details, names, and minutiae. Better still, my problem-solving ability was increased. The difficulty of academic challenges paled noticeably. I was able to devise experiments that were both complex and elegant to arrive at my scientific endpoints. In short, improved fitness proved critical to being a better scientist.

As Edison famously said, "Genius is 1 percent inspiration and 99 percent perspiration." The betterment of my brain would largely have been wasted if I hadn't exerted myself to carry out the experiments I thought up. Science is slow work, full of blind alleys. Without a lot of effort, even the smartest person's progress can be reduced to a crawl. Naturally, I had much more energy as a result of my diet and exercise regimen, and I was able to apply my newfound stamina to my research. I would work late into the night most days of the week to complete experiments, and then go exercise. This constant effort, combined with more than a little good luck, propelled me to one of the quicker graduations our program had seen in recent times. By the time my dissertation defense arrived, I had a plethora of scientific achievements on my resumé, including published scientific articles, presentations at major research conferences, and the filing of several patents. Only a fraction of this would have been possible if I had gone through graduate school in my previous poor physical and mental condition. Never was this change exemplified more than at the finish, as I was able to turn on the afterburners to prepare for a major academic event the day after a gigantic race. I doubt I would have even had the confidence to attempt something this ambitious as little as a year previously. In the immediate sense, the rewards were coming rapidly, but the payoff began only after a long sequence of efforts.

Finishing my PhD was of paramount importance to me for the same reason conquering physical challenges were. There are precious few things you can invest in that cannot be taken away arbitrarily: education, personal experiences, your body, and the relationships you form. With the exception of physical health, which I had only recently embraced, I had always pursued these "permanent" investments as long-term, high-priority goals. As a character issue, finishing something I had started was also quite important for me in and of itself. One of the principles I have emphasized, particularly in racing and academics, is not quitting. Even though I was somewhat miserable, I finished my undergraduate program. And even though I was sometimes reduced to walking, I would finish every race I entered. Sometimes, all it takes to succeed is simply carrying on.

Now was by no means a time to rest on my laurels. Merely having a final defense scheduled was no guarantee of receiving a degree. Months earlier, a student in my program had run into some trouble and was delayed for months in graduating, and it was not unheard of for senior students to fail outright. Out of the 300 million or so people in the United States, only about five thousand earn doctorates in medical research every year.[14] For my attempt, I would be presenting my research findings in a public talk, followed by a longer question-and-answer session with the four tenured professors of my thesis committee. That would be the hard part. Their decision on whether I was good enough to join their ranks, on the basis of my presentation and the quality of my answers in subsequent discussion, was final. Getting through the entire ordeal was never a given, and I made my final preparations with this in mind.

My mother had arrived to watch the proceedings, and I was quickly exhausted from trying to entertain my parents, putting the final touches on my presentation, and keeping my cool under pressure. Scientific presentations, even at the highest levels, have a rich tradition of being done at the very last second, and I was hardly one to buck a trend. The night before the dissertation defense was scheduled, I dragged my parents into the lab so I could take some photos of cells I wanted to talk about the following morning.

I needn't have troubled myself with my eleventh-hour efforts. The talk went smoothly, and the members of my committee were more inquisitive than antagonistic. I had collected the requisite signatures to approve the conferral of my degree less than three hours after I began. Almost exactly four years earlier, I had been morbidly obese and had barely managed to scrape through a bachelor's program. In the past three days, I had won a spot at the national triathlon championships and earned a PhD with flying colors. If I hadn't been there for both of these events, I wouldn't have believed it myself.

# Chicago

---

*"Smooth seas do not make skillful sailors."*
—AFRICAN PROVERB

On March 10th, 2007, I drove away from Gainesville for the last time, to begin the next phase of my professional life. During my final days at the University of Florida, I had been proactive in searching for what would be the first "real" job in my life. It was an interesting experience. A job search in academia is similar in many ways to trying to get a girlfriend in middle school. Both processes are generally initiated with a series of introductory notes, followed by a mutual checking of references. If all goes well, this is followed by an awkward phone conversation in which a fine line is walked between appearing too nonchalant and too desperate. And, of course, both endeavors carry a significant risk of personal rejection.

I had narrowed a long list of laboratories down to two prospective employers: Dr. Mark Mattson at the National Institute of Aging and Dr. Bruce Lahn at the University of Chicago. Both were stellar scientists, but I was particularly fascinated with Dr. Mattson's work. It was Mark who, years before, had authored the very study on intermittent fasting that I had appropriated for my weight-loss experiment. I arranged a meeting with him, and soon thereafter I was on a plane to visit his laboratory in Baltimore.

Mark was well known in the scientific community for advocating the argument that caloric restriction was a valid method for dramatically extending lifespan and improving long-term health. When I met him, it was immediately evident that he practiced what he preached. Mark had the physique of an elite marathoner: he was five-foot-ten and weighed no more than 130 pounds. At lunch, Mark selected only a mini bagel and two small apples. I watched, grimly fascinated, as he hungrily devoured every last morsel, including cores and stems, in a matter of seconds. Sitting there with no evidence of having ever eaten, Mark watched me eat my own lunch, his eyes alertly tracking the fork as it traversed the gulf between plate and mouth. I left the meeting a little freaked out. Though I had great respect for the work Mark had done, I found his approach to portion control a little extreme for my tastes—too much (or too little, actually) of a good thing.

My subsequent experience at the University of Chicago proved a little more normal. Dr. Lahn's lab was one of only several hundred funded by the ultra-exclusive Howard Hughes Medical Institute. Working there would provide me an unusually high level of job security and funding relative to most postdoc positions, not to mention access to the most cutting-edge tools. The research group was full of smart, friendly people. I followed my instincts and signed on the dotted line less than a week later.

Like most things in my life in those days, the move to my new job happened more quickly than I would have liked. After finishing the years-long process of earning a doctorate, it's typical to take some time off to decompress and leisurely ponder the next phase of your career. I, however, after completing my dissertation defense, took the rest of the afternoon off before returning to pick up where I'd left off in the lab. There I remained until the day before I was scheduled to leave town. I had given myself two days to drive to Chicago before beginning work the following Monday. Just to make sure I didn't get too much rest on the drive up, I scheduled a detour through Jacksonville, where I jumped out of the car and ran my final Gate River Run as a Florida resident. Like my running pace, my life had dramatically accelerated as well.

As someone who has devoted large amounts of time studying the brain, I am always amazed by how many daily life decisions are made through entirely unconscious mechanisms, a sort of autopilot for the brain. It was somewhat ironic then, that I began to do a little thinking after kicking the car into cruise control for the thousand-mile trip to Chicago. I was thinking not about where I'd been, but about where I was going. Having spent slightly less than two days in Chicago before deciding to move there, I was heading into essentially unknown territory. After my initial visit, I hadn't bothered to come back to find an apartment, instead deciding to save a little on airfare by rolling the dice on finding something through the internet.

In fact, since Chicago was on Lake Michigan, I thought it would be cool to live on a houseboat, just like MacGyver. Yet I couldn't seem to find any listings. Finally, someone told me there were no houseboats to be had because Lake Michigan was frozen over five months out of the year. This was the first sign I might be getting more than I'd bargained for. Roommates from hell or a bedroom the size of a broom closet could be worked around; weather and urban sprawl were less flexible entities. I had an Ironman in a month, and I was beginning to realize the consequences of the fact that I would be completing the final phase of preparation in one of the most urban environments in the United States, on the tail end of the vicious Chicago winter. According to the Weather Channel's website, the average temperatures in Chicago and Anchorage, Alaska, differ by only a few degrees during winter and early spring. The thin blood of a southerner ran through my veins, and winter in Florida amounted to little more than an opportunity to break out my lone pair of jeans. As I entered Indiana, I began to see the first traces of snow and ice and lamented not investing in a bit more winter weather gear before blindly heading north.

My trepidation increased with each passing mile. At the Indiana-Illinois border I passed the industrial cesspool of Gary, Indiana, and found I was depressingly close to my new home, which was in Hyde Park, the neighborhood that surrounds the University of Chicago. Hyde Park is a famous old neighborhood (my apartment hailed from the nineteenth century), a former bastion of the rich abattoir owners from Chicago's bygone days as a meatpacking center. Despite its formerly high standing, the neighborhood had long since been engulfed by urban sprawl, and was now surrounded by some significantly lower-income neighborhoods. My directions had taken me off the interstate a little early, so I was treated to an impromptu and very frightening tour of the Chicago ghetto as I approached from the south. I locked the doors as I rolled past groups of men sitting on ramshackle porches, drinking forty-ounce containers of malt liquor at 9:30 in the morning. My foot hovered over the accelerator, ready to floor it should anyone discharge a firearm in my direction. Somehow, I hadn't been shown this part of town on my initial visit. Less than three blocks away from my new address, I was already caressing my cell phone, ready to call Florida and beg for my old job back. Suddenly, the neighborhood dramatically changed. I had reached Hyde Park.

So long as I stayed within the one square mile of the neighborhood, I appeared to be relatively safe. The neighborhood was rigidly defined, bordered on the east by Lake Michigan and on the west by Washington Park, the proposed site of the Olympic stadium in the city's bid for the 2016 summer games. According to my research, the park and the lakefront were among the better places to run and bike. I decided to begin my reconnaissance of the area by foot, along the lakefront path. However, I became directionally confused and ran in the opposite direction, inland to Washington Park. Given the Olympian status that the park aspired to, I was expecting something a little more impressive than the giant featureless pasture that greeted me. An uneven gravel jogging track surrounded acres of listless grass. I decided to run a few laps and get the lay of the land. I had run about half a loop when a group of teenage girls flagged me down. They wanted me to take a picture with them; I was the first white person they had seen jogging in the park in some time. I later learned that, in spite of the city's significant populations of African-American, Hispanic, Polish, and Asian heritage, the neighborhoods in Chicago remained largely segregated. Washington Park lay just outside the boundary of mostly white Hyde Park. Racial differences didn't bother me, and the park seemed more dead than dangerous, so I shrugged it off and continued exploring.

On my second lap of the park, I wasn't asked for photos or autographs, but something even more bizarre happened. As I rounded the southernmost corner of the jogging path, a parrot suddenly fluttered to a landing in front of me. Perplexed, I stopped. The bird gave me a cursory once-over, strutted to the edge of the path, and began pecking at a patch of snow nonchalantly. I'll say it again: a parrot, in Chicago, in March, landed on the ground and pecked at the snow. Several questions occurred to me, the most pressing of which was whether I was seeing or imagining this. I was quickly able to rule out a mirage. The day was cool, if not brutally cold. The next most likely explanation was that someone had misplaced the family pet. As quickly as it occurred to me, the escaped-pet theory was dashed as an almost identical parrot swooped in, landing a few feet from the first and clucking happily. With legitimate explanations for this surreal vision dwindling, I did what any astute man of science would do: I got the hell out of there. Later than night, from the safety of my apartment, I did a web search on the presence of wild parrots in Chicago, praying that my next search would not be for a good therapist. I hit pay dirt almost immediately: there was indeed a population of feral monk parrots (no doubt originally introduced by careless homeowners) that had colonized the area surrounding Washington Park since the early 1970s. All of this was just too surreal for me. I could easily handle being the only white guy in a one-mile radius, but there is simply no way to prepare yourself for seeing parrots in the midst of a winter snowstorm.

Hoping for a less alarming experience, I decided to try my luck next on the pedestrian path that runs through Chicago along Lake Michigan. I lived only half a mile from the lake, and the route promised to be far more scenic than the track in Washington Park. I cruised past the sprawling Museum of Science and Industry, the lone original building remaining on the site of the 1893 World's Fair, and passed through a tunnel underneath the ten lanes of Lake Shore Drive. After ascending one final ramp, I was suddenly a stone's throw away from the choppy gray-blue waters of Lake Michigan. There was a choice to make: I could run either north, toward downtown Chicago, or south, toward the Indiana border. Since I could see clouds of industrial smog emanating from the not-so-distant smokestacks of Gary, I chose to go north, where the air was flavored by less sinister forms of pollution. Chicago's well-deserved nickname, "The Windy City," ostensibly originates from its contentious political past, but it's also an homage to the unyielding and often forceful winds coming off the lake all year long. This day was colder than the previous one, and though it was overcast, the winds were as gusty as ever. Even while sheltered by inland buildings, I could feel it blowing and swirling, a mere hint of what I would face when I was fully exposed to its fury. Braced to encounter the brunt of Chicago's winter wrath, I emerged by the lake proper. It was a pleasant surprise, then, when I found myself cruising along unmolested. The path was made of smooth asphalt, flanked by gravel shoulders for sore-kneed joggers, and was in a far better state of repair than its Washington Park counterpart. Despite the ideal location and design, the path was essentially deserted. Why was no one out there? As time passed, I became increasingly aware that

I wasn't merely running—I was *flying* along, and doing so with only a minimal expenditure of effort.

And then I turned around.

It had never occurred to me that the reason I was running so well was not my natural ability, but the fact that I was propelled by a constant 30-mile-per-hour breeze at my back. Oh. My. God. When I attempted to go in the opposite direction, it felt as though I had run directly into an ice-cold invisible wall. My speed was literally cut in half as I was reduced to a miserable imitation of jogging. My testicles ascended into my body, seeking warmth, but no such option existed for my other extremities. My ungloved hands froze, assuming the form of twisted claws. My right contact lens iced up and made a bid to escape, and my creepy hobble was made even more repulsive by a perpetual compensatory wink. For the second time in two days, I seriously considered calling the whole thing off and moving back to Florida, where I didn't have to worry about my internal fluids thickening into sludge from the cold. It was a scenario I might well have enacted, but for the lack of strength in my frozen hands to unlock and start my car.

The wind was but one of Chicago's meteorological quirks. I discovered another curiosity of the local weather the very next weekend. In the midst of the city's annual St. Patrick's Day Parade, snow began to fall. Normally, this would not bear mentioning, but this snowstorm was remarkable, as the snow fell from a sky innocent of any clouds. With my primitive understanding of the origins of precipitation, I believed this to be something of an impossibility. More internet research netted me the following explanation: because of the highly differential temperatures of relatively warm water and arctic air currents, coupled with orographic lift, there exists in leeward landmasses adjacent to substantive bodies of water a propensity for localized precipitation. To nonmeteorologists, this means that it can snow along the lake with little or no warning. Locals call this "lake-effect snow," but generally have no idea, in my experience, as to what the term actually means. Taking advantage of this bit of ignorance, I began using "lake effect" as an excuse for everything: a bad hair day, the political situation in Iraq, a failed experiment, etc. Most people seemed to be OK with this, absorbing my utterance with a serious-looking nod and accepting its veracity at face value.

Human beings are nothing if not adaptable to new circumstances, and I eventually made the necessary adjustments to conduct outdoor activities in my new neck of the woods. Most of these adjustments involved wearing both more and increasingly elaborate types of clothing. I swam in the university pool, a beautiful (and heated) indoor facility. As the weeks passed, the weather reluctantly improved and my training became largely unhampered by the elements. Similar to preparing for running races, a key feature of my training plan was a long multisport workout every weekend, with a final massive effort close to the actual race distance a few weeks before the competition. Then I would rest, letting my body build its capacities back up for the event itself. My last big day before the Ironman was planned to consist of eighty miles of biking and twenty-two miles of running, spread out over several workouts throughout the day. But Mother Nature chose this day to break out a new type of confounding weather phenomenon: a pea-soup fog that rolled in before dawn and refused to burn off. If the lake effect made it snow, what the hell was the reason for this? This was one mystery I never unraveled.

As I stepped out the front door I felt like I'd gone to bed in Chicago and woken up in London. Running was surrealistic; people and landmarks would appear and disappear in the fog like ghosts. The fog was too dense to let me safely navigate a bike, so I spent over four hours riding a stationary bike, which is not recommended for children, women who are nursing, or anyone else, for that matter. Then it was back into the mist, which was really starting to remind me of the Stephen King novella of the same name. Literally my whole day was spent exercising, good practice for what was in store. Toward the end of the run, I was, naturally enough, getting rather tired. In order to squeeze the last two or three miles out of my legs, I deliberately ran into a very seedy neighborhood, figuring that the motivation of avoiding potential muggers would help me keep going. I managed to pull that particular trick off, but I still ponder whether this was a brilliant or foolhardy maneuver—I was so tired and weak that a gang of seven-year-olds could have defeated me at that point.

Speaking of thugs, it bears mentioning that my training grounds on the south side of Chicago were home to a substantial amount of gang activity. On colder days, I had come to favor wearing a bandana on my head to stay warm and keep sweat out of my eyes. After wearing a blue bandana on a few runs, I noticed that I was getting some incredulous looks each time I ventured south of Hyde Park. I asked around and discovered I had inadvertently been running through one gang's turf while wearing the colors of one of their rivals. It was fortunate that I managed to navigate the streets for as long as I did without serious incident. Unwilling to give up wearing a bandana altogether, I cast about for a new color that was gang-neutral. I discovered I had two options whose safety was ironclad: pink or some earth tone.

Alas, they don't make taupe bandanas.

# The Flight into Danger

*The attainment of wholeness requires one
to stake one's whole being. Nothing less will
do; there can be no easier conditions, no
substitutes, no compromises.*

—CARL JUNG

It was go time. My period of rest and recovery had flown by in the blink of an eye, taken up by new projects at work and my explorations of the nicer (and less dangerous) parts of Chicago. The lead-up to Ironman Arizona was interesting for another reason: I almost won a race. Sort of. One weekend during my rest period, I had driven uptown to get in a short jog, just to keep my legs in shape. By coincidence, a race was in progress in the area where I was jogging: the Chicago Lakefront 50K, an ultramarathon race. While most races have closed courses, this race was in such a high-traffic location that the organizers had to allow casual runners to mix in with the racers. Long-distance runners are generally a mellow group of people, and I enjoyed running amongst them. Naturally, I was running faster than most everyone, as my legs were still fresh and springy, and I passed from one group of racers to another, saying a positive word and moving on. By the halfway point of my run, the participants had thinned out, until it was clear that I was near the front of the race. I passed one guy who responded with a surge of his own. Neither of us was wearing a race number, which meant we were both casual runners. This was bad etiquette on his part; once passed, a runner should not immediately re-pass. It's an unwritten rule in recreational running, and I got a little irked. *OK, buddy, you wanna play? Let's do it.* I returned the surge, drawing ahead. For good measure, I gave it a little extra speed, just to punish the guy for showing such machismo on a casual run.

I was running too fast for my own good, but I had made my point, having established a little cushion between myself and my would-be competitor. Coming around one of the gentle bends in the trail, I caught sight of the finish for the race. Upon seeing us both, the small but vocal crowd began hooting and hollering. A finish tape was threaded across the path. Something wasn't right. I took a quick glance at the chuffing runner struggling to catch up to me. There it was: a pared-down race number pinned to his shorts on the leg I couldn't see. I had just passed one of the top finishers, maybe even the leader. Seeing us both running so hard, the crowd naturally assumed we were engaged in a sprint to the finish.

Racing during training is poor form. Winning a race you're not participating in takes it to a whole new level. I had already tortured the poor guy needlessly (if inadvertently); there was no way I could break the tape first. For the first time in my life, I needed to lose ground, and fast. Like a professional wrestler, I immediately feigned an injury. I stopped so fast, it must have looked like I was shot by a sniper. As I pretended to hobble, my "competitor" gained on me, but slowly. It was going to be close. With only seconds to spare, he passed me, seemingly pulling off a dramatic victory.

I passed through the finish a moment later. There was nowhere else to go, no side path to take. Despite having no idea who I was, several people yelled out that I had made a great effort. I had two options: stay and pretend I was in the race (and possibly be presented with an award) or keep going. I was seriously worried about being attacked for inadvertently deceiving everyone, so I decided to punch it and make a break while the crowd was still disorganized. My limp disappeared, and I got the hell out of there even faster than I had arrived. "Where ya' goin'?" I heard, as I scampered away. There was no time to answer. There was a real race to run next week, and real hobbling to do.

Early Wednesday morning of race week, I rose uncomfortably early and endured a bleary-eyed hour on the elevated train to O'Hare Airport for the flight to Phoenix. After giving some forethought to how functional my body would be after the punishment I was asking it to absorb, I had packed a bare minimum of gear. My possessions fit into a single backpack, which contained both equipment for racing and civilian clothes. I had chosen to ship my bike to the race site, where it would be assembled and ready for pickup when I arrived, so I wasn't even checking a bag. As the big day approached, I had become increasingly worried about a last-minute injury or ailment screwing everything up and had begun treating my body as though it were as fragile as an infant's. On the flight, I was popping up compulsively every twenty minutes to stretch my legs. No deep-vein thrombosis for me! I was rewarded for my frequent stirring by arriving at Phoenix Sky-Harbor Airport whole and healthy. The first order of business was to rendezvous with my father and Jen, who had flown all the way from North Carolina and Florida to support me. Walking out of the terminal, I experienced heat shock, which was not altogether unpleasant. I was still dressed for Chicago, which was a full forty degrees cooler than the sunny and cloudless day that greeted us. I had expected to encounter weather of this sort, going so far as to spend time in the sauna during periods of recovery from training in an attempt to acclimate myself to dry, hot conditions. Despite these special preparations, I still needed to make a big adjustment to the Phoenix weather, which was like night and day compared to the foggy, windy icebox I had been training in. There was nothing I could do about it at this point but hope that my early arrival would help me adapt to the local climate. At least I'd get my tan back.

We had rented a car for the week, and the drive from the airport afforded us our first look at the greater Phoenix/Tempe area. It seemed like a cheerful place, a medium-sized college town home to Arizona State University. The next item on the agenda was registering at the race site, which, in true testament to the organizers at North American Sports, was far from the chaotic free-for-all I had anticipated. This was my first exposure to an Ironman race and the athletes who participate in them. The competitors were pretty easy to spot: they were the extremely lean, extremely muscular people strolling around in old running shoes and sporting well-worn t-shirts from other triathlons. Everyone looked a little too serious and a lot too nervous, considering that the race was still a full four days away. At the weigh-in, I came in at 205 pounds, slightly more than I'd expected but not entirely inexplicable. Training for a triathlon altered my body composition in ways that no single sport did. Although my outward appearance had changed very little, I had become super-dense from the added muscle mass in my waist and upper body, as well as adept at retaining large amounts of fluid to sweat out as needed. I was literally in the best shape of my life, and what the scale said wasn't terribly important at that point. Besides, I had a feeling that a lot of my water weight would be gone within a couple of days.

The next day, I dragged my entourage back to race headquarters. The swim course had been opened for practice, and it had been a while since I'd had the opportunity to swim in open water. I'd hoped to avail myself of Lake Michigan, but I thought I saw chunks of ice in the water up until the day I left. Tempe Town Lake, Tempe's main body of water, was host to the swim portion of the event. The lake was actually a man-made canal that was shaped in a long, narrow rectangle. The water didn't look so healthy, but I was assured it was safe enough. I squeezed into my trusty wetsuit and popped in for a quick dip. In the following forty minutes I was exposed as the bad swimmer I truly was by the flocks of competitors who flew by and left me in their wake. Over and over, I was passed by groups, single swimmers, and (I could have sworn) a couple of people with only one arm. It was clear I wasn't going to be winning the swim portion of this competition. But this concerned me little. Swimming remained my weakest discipline of the three. It was a logical decision to leave it that way, and one easy to validate. The relatively short length of the swim compared to the rest of the triathlon (especially at the Iron-man level) made swimming less of a priority for an amateur athlete like me. As a result, I was competent but hardly spectacular. To compensate for my lack of speed, I had become proficient at swimming tactically. I would closely follow other, faster swimmers, which provided a reduction in drag and thus a boost in velocity, if done correctly. This technique, called drafting, was both legal and a great equalizer for weaker swimmers. During that day's practice, as yet another swimmer passed me, I shifted over to take advantage of his draft. I lost him almost immediately; he was too speedy even to cling to like the swimming parasite I was. Climbing back onto dry land, I resigned myself to having a long day in the water.

The swim segment of the race was to be a single loop of almost two-and-a-half miles. I'd never even seen a swim course that large, much less swum one. My little practice swim hadn't taken me far enough to even see the midpoint of that distance, so I did a short run on the path alongside the lake (also part of the run course) to find the end of this rainbow. I had to run pretty damn far before I found the turnaround. Looking down the bank of the lake, it was impossible to see the six-foot-high turnaround buoy from the start point.

My official business concluded for the day, I suggested we go to lunch. In spite of their tough image, endurance athletes can be babies about some things, and right now I needed to be fed. While my father was also ready to eat, Jen begged for a postponement. She had visited the race expo earlier, and the vendors, eager to cater to a pretty girl, had fallen over themselves to feed her various high-energy foodstuffs. To kill a few minutes, we climbed to the top of a small but steep hill in the middle of Tempe which provided my sherpas a superb panoramic view of the swim course. "You're going to swim that?" my dad said, looking through the zoom lens of my camera at the turnaround in the distance, and tracing the course back to the start. "Good luck. I'll be eating free granola at the expo with Jen. Call if you need a ride back."

The following day, after another poor swimming demonstration by yours truly, we inspected the bike course in our rental car. The route was set up as three equal loops of approximately forty miles each. Each circuit began in the middle of town, then headed northeast on the Beeline highway, through the Salt River Indian community. The outbound section of each lap concluded with a gradual climb of eight miles before returning to town on the same road. No fewer than a dozen crazed competitors were riding the forty-mile loop in the baking sun just two days before the race. I silently toasted each of them with a Diet Coke as I conserved my resources from within the air-conditioned comfort of our rental car. Just because you're fit or tough (or both) doesn't mean you're smart.

Tempe did have one thing in common with Chicago: wind, and lots of it. A small sandstorm blew through town on Friday night, covering my bike in a fine grit that required painstaking removal. On Saturday morning, I placed the gear I would need to navigate the transitions between the race segments into two bags provided for that purpose and deposited them, along with my now-sparkling bike, at the main transition zone at race headquarters. With nothing left to practice, tweak, or clean before the actual race, I became utterly infantile, unwilling to tire out my legs to even the slightest degree by walking around or even standing around for extended periods. Jen and my father were sweet enough to accommodate my delicacy, so we went to the movies and

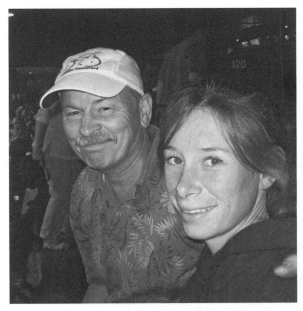

**Jennifer and Dad, both glad they're not the ones racing tomorrow.**

then to a baseball game, where I ate ballpark peanuts and a turkey sub the night before the biggest race of my life.

Later, I lay in bed and thought about where I'd been and where I was going. In particular, I reconsidered the training adage that getting to the starting line of a race was its own reward. Considering how long it had taken me to get there, I had to agree. True to form for the day, I slept like a baby.

# Ironman

*If God invented marathons to keep people
from doing anything more stupid, the
Ironman must have taken Him completely
by surprise.*

—P.Z. PEARCE

To some degree, the routine on the morning before every big race re-
calls the movie *Groundhog Day*, a tightly regimented but panicked comedy. The details are a little different each time, but, ultimately, the story
always winds up in the same place. It's still dark outside when the wake-
up call snaps you out of a fitful dream. Apprehension blooms: phone
calls that can't wait until you've had a cup of coffee rarely offer good
news. Suddenly, the purpose of the call is remembered and you're fully
alert. Just enough adrenaline trickles into your bloodstream to make
you shiver in the cool, sterile air of the hotel room, and the barely noticeable taste of nervous stomach acid invades the back of your throat.
Going back to sleep, even at four in the morning, is no longer a possibility. Organizational thoughts arrive and depart in no apparent order.
Find the bathroom. Get dressed. Eat something. Not too much. Drink
lots of Gatorade. Where the hell is the bathroom? If you're sick or hurt
today, it's all over. You test every joint and muscle to make sure they're
working the same as when you went to bed, and each little creak and
snap warrants far more attention than it would on any other day. In the

cracks in your routine, chaos dwells, and you can't help but engage in the most pointless activity: worrying whether you've prepared enough to pull off what you're about to try. The alarm is the first beginning, setting you on a well-trodden path that ends where the race begins. The starting cannon is the second beginning, blasting away your stewing apprehension and the familiarity of routine. No matter how long or how many times you've prepared, every race is at least a little different, and you have no earthly idea what to expect.

I drove with my father and Jen through the streets of Tempe, deserted at this early hour, arriving in plenty of time to make the start. Even so, we were among the last arrivals. An orderly mob had filled every space around the race start site, as though it were totally normal for five thousand people to be milling around at 5:00 AM. The obsessive type-A triathletes were on full display. I overheard one woman say she'd been up since 3:00 AM and still felt a little rushed. Like me, virtually every competitor had a support crew, but most seemed unaware of their entourage, more concerned with battling their own demons as the starting time loomed. At this late hour, all the preparations either had happened or weren't going to, and there was little left to do. I prepped my bike, made one last check of my stored consumables, and found a peaceful-looking rock to sit on. My father had drifted off for the moment, soaking up the energy and excitement of the pre-race atmosphere. Jen sat, shivering, with me as I suckled Gatorade, trying to leech away my body heat in the cool pre-dawn darkness. As the first rays of the cresting sun peeked over the desert, the public address system crackled to life, calling first professionals, then amateurs, into the water. I pulled my wetsuit over my shoulders, downed one last energy gel to top off the gas tank, and, like a child in need of reassurance, solicited a hug from my father and Jen. "This'll just take a second. We'll do lunch after," I joked, joining the long queue of shuffling, neoprene-clad athletes.

The atmosphere was more apprehensive than eager. There was little conversation as we clambered over the lake's retaining wall and onto a dock. Some competitors had progressed from suitably nervous to plain scared, and I saw tears on more than one face. We had to jump off the dock into the reservoir, and I couldn't help but notice that there was no way to climb back out—the only avenue of escape was the steps at the swim finish. I felt numb as I dog-paddled to the swim start. The motions of swimming suddenly felt foreign and unfamiliar to me. I remembered that race officials had mentioned to us earlier in the week that more than half of the people in the field were doing their first Ironman. Why was that? The most likely explanation I could muster was that only a fraction of people who had done the race once were dumb or brave enough to try another. Why hadn't this occurred to me earlier and why was I thinking about it now? I tried to push that nasty little thought from my mind as I treaded water.

In order for all 2,100 competitors to start simultaneously, race organizers started us from within the deep water of the lake, rather than from a beach. Hundreds of heads bobbed around me, alternately moving up and down like the world's largest game of bop-a-mole. At ten 'til 7:00, the sixty-three professional athletes in the field began their race. As they streamed away at a preternatural speed, the race director shifted his energies to motivating the amateur triathletes and the crowd that lined the lake's retaining walls and overhead bridges. "You're going to be an IRONMAN today!" he exulted, his proclamation met by frenetic cheering from all assembled. I conserved my huzzah, saving all my energy for later in the day. I had optimistically positioned myself a couple of rows behind the vanguard, hoping to find a good pair of feet to pace myself off of for as long as possible. With no preparatory countdown, the starting cannon went off abruptly. I clicked my watch to start the timer and embarked on the first of 140.6 miles.

The mass start of an Ironman is a treat to behold, if not to experience. After it was all over, Jen showed me some video she had taken of the start. From a safe distance, it looked downright placid: swimmers moved gracefully through the water on effortlessly pinwheeling arms, while cheers from the spectators ebbed and flowed, with the U2 song "Beautiful Day" playing in the background. "Make some noise," the announcer urged the crowd. "They can hear you!" The only thing I could hear was my heart pounding against my ribcage and the regular whooshing of my arms entering the water. The urgent need for air hit me in short intervals. As I broke water to draw deep, ragged breaths, the splashing sound from the packed humanity surrounding me gave the impression that I was swimming through a waterfall. My existence was distilled to a simple recipe. Four strokes. Breathe. Repeat as needed. Precious little pierced my bubble of sensory deprivation. Time ceased to have meaning, estimated only by the rate at which the passing scenery changed. Distance perception was also lost. Occasionally, my personal space was challenged, as were my manners. Just as important as swimming forward is avoiding the sometimes devastating collisions that occur when too many people are packed into too little water. Near the turnaround point, I was reminded that swimming could be a contact sport when an elbow clocked me solidly on the side of my head. Colorful stars were still parading across my field of vision minutes later.

The trip back was arduous. Between the head injury and mediocre swim skills, I was not having a good day in the water. It felt as though I was swimming in place. I had spotted the bridge that marked the finish, but I wasn't getting any closer. It was the reverse of a desert mirage, where I was already in the water but couldn't get out. Lost in that thought, I was surprised by the abrupt left turn to the swim exit. After that, we faced a final two hundred meters across a narrow channel, concluding on a wide set of carpeted steps. Reaching the stairs, I grabbed a rail and tried to pull myself out of the water, but my legs flatly refused to support me. Whether this was a lingering effect of the shot to the head or a severe case of jelly legs after an absurdly long swim, if I didn't stand up, I was going to get run over and likely drown in eight inches of water. The second attempt at recapturing a bipedal stature proved more successful, and I lurched forward amid the rubber-capped crowd of transitioning swimmers.

As I regained my equilibrium, I removed my swim cap and was not terribly surprised to find that it contained blood from my ear's brief encounter with a strange elbow. As I turned the corner, I was confronted by a phalanx of wetsuit strippers, volunteers whose sole purpose was to assist racers in rapidly removing their skintight wetsuits. One such individual ordered me to lie down on my back in the tone of an exasperated mother that who would brook no argument. Having worked rather hard to stand so recently, I was reluctant to cede my gains in balance. Before I could adequately explain this, she had seized my wetsuit at the shoulders, and I was left with no choice but to comply. I sat down, straightened my legs and pointed my toes, and she whipped my suit off with the flair of a magician pulling a tablecloth off a bedecked four-top. I struggled back to my feet and collected my wetsuit, marveling at the speed and efficiency of the technique. As I rejoined the half-walking/half-jogging throng, a flash of pale white buttock caught my eye. The guy next to me was not wearing the bike shorts most of us sported underneath our wetsuits. Initially, I thought he was completely naked, but a second glance revealed him to be clad in a zebra-print thong that left nothing to the imagination. All I could think of was that this guy's wetsuit stripper must have inadvertently ripped his shorts off in the process of removing his wetsuit. I wondered what the etiquette was for saying something. This thought was followed by the stomach-sinking realization that I had undergone an identical procedure, and I was not 100 percent certain that I was still clad in bike shorts myself. This could be problematic; I had opted to race unthonged. For all I knew, people were laughing at both of us as we paraded past. I glanced down, almost tripping over my wetsuit in the process, but managed to verify that both my shorts and my modesty were safely preserved.

The transition zone was a cheerful chaos managed by an army of harried volunteers. I grabbed my bag of supplies, sat down as far away as possible from Manthongamus Prime (who, I noted, had complemented the fashion statement with dual nipple rings), and slipped on my socks, shoes, helmet, and race number. On steadying legs, I proceeded to the bike area, where a smiling volunteer was waiting with my bike and a wish for a smooth ride. I was in and out in less time than it took to pick up dinner at a drive-through.

My body felt good and my spirits were high as I started the mammoth 112-mile bike segment. My swim and first transition put me smack in the middle of the field, as good as I could have hoped for. I had given some thought to setting time goals, but the overwhelming majority of opinions from race veterans encouraged me to keep my focus on simply finishing. That sounded perfectly reasonable to me as I pedaled through downtown Tempe and into the Sonoran desert. The day was turning predictably hot, and the few wispy clouds floating in the bright blue sky failed to shield me from the sun's wrath. I wistfully thought back to the sunscreen station I had bypassed in transition with the thought of saving a few seconds, but twelve-plus hours in the sun were going to break down any SPF this side of 500 anyway. Ten short miles into the bike segment, it was clear that I would not be sleeping on my back that night.

I had established a nice rhythm, and I hit the turnaround for the first loop in about an hour. Most of the bike route was outside of the city limits, in the barren desolation of the mesa desert. Outside of town, the only people we saw were aid station volunteers. After the crowding of the swim, the packs of athletes had thinned out and I increasingly found myself alone, with only the roadside armies of silent cacti for company.

No matter how fast you are on a bike, covering such a huge distance requires hours and hours of time. Even though the act of pedaling a bike in a straight line requires less brainpower than tying a shoe, a surprising number of things kept me busy. Like all good triathletes, I was engrossed with executing my plan and reacting to the changing conditions in the race and in my body. Months before, I had watched the broadcast of the previous year's race and noted how the announcers stressed the need to stay fueled and hydrated. Keeping fed and watered was my number one priority for the bike portion of the event. I was carrying energy gels and bars, as well as water and Gatorade, constantly evaluating how much fluid and how many calories I should consume to keep myself going. I had to walk a fine line: consume too little and I would suffer the lethargy from an energy drain; consume too much and I would begin to bloat and get an upset stomach. It was critical that I listen to my body, something I had gotten pretty good at by now. Just as important as the food and drink, I was regularly consuming salt tablets to replace the electrolytes I lost through sweat. These would keep me from cramping up later in the day.

It was also important to continue monitoring my progress. This means different things to different people, depending on your goals at the beginning of the race, including your overall position in the race, your placing compared to others in your age group, and your overall time. Nowhere was this chess match more apparent than at the front of the pack of racers. As I headed out on my first loop, I began to see the leading professionals go past in the opposite direction, streaking along at a speed more evocative of jets than of bicycles. Even though it was early in the game, it was evident that each pro's attention was on a razor's edge. Each face was taught with tension, each biker alert and ready to respond to the moves of his competitors, or perhaps make his own move if he sensed weakness. Decisions made now would be proven right or wrong only hours later, and both day and strategy wore on. I felt a newfound respect for the mental demands of a sport known mostly for the physical ones.

While most sports are played in a controlled environment, triathlons are sprawling affairs that introduce the variables of terrain and weather. Today, the weather had begun to announce itself as a major factor in the equation. By the halfway point of the first loop of the bike segment, the wind had increased steadily and was blowing directly against riders on the return to town. In spite of a downhill slope, cyclists pedaling into the wind appeared to be navigating through some sort of reverse gravity. As we came back into the city limits, the crowds reappeared. I spotted my father and Jen in the crowd outside race headquarters and gave them a big thumbs-up to signal that I was OK. Starting the second lap, I hit the no-man's-land of the middle miles of the Ironman and began to have my first problems of the day.

I was still riding the same entry-level road bike I'd first started on in North Carolina. Although bikes designed specifically for triathlons exist, mine had served me well to this point, and I possessed neither the means nor the inclination to buy a more specialized piece of equipment. But by my fourth hour on the Ironman Arizona bike course, I was beginning to regret not forking out the jack for a proper triathlon bike. My road bike was nimble and maneuverable, good for riding in groups, but a triathlon bike would have put me in a more comfortable, wind-friendly position, increasing my aerodynamics (i.e., giving me free speed) at the expense of handling. Since the rules forbade me from sheltering myself in the slipstreams of other riders, I was having to work harder than I would have on a better bike to maintain the same speed. The winds had intensified during the day, reaching speeds high enough to warrant a closure of the airport, for the safety of multi-ton commercial jets. No such reprieve was granted to the racers, and I cursed my skinflint nature as the day wore on. The return portion of the second loop was very difficult. Sweat stung my eyes and ran down my nose, pinging against my bike's frame.

The extra expenditure of energy was sapping me. The caloric requirements to finish an Ironman are mind-boggling. Completing the event required in excess of ten thousand calories, enough energy to power five normal people for an entire day. On each loop of the bike course I consumed two 32-ounce bottles of Gatorade, two 20-ounce water bottles, two energy bars, and two energy gels. Over three laps, this would add up to 3,300 calories. Every bit of this, and then some, would be completely burned for fuel. I was actually going through calories faster than I could take them in. The difference came out of my body's stores of energy, of which there was a finite supply. The trick was to push myself as hard as I dared without actually running out of gas too far from the finish line.

My headway through the gale was slow, and the baking sun and ample time worked in concert to elicit some odd thoughts. I began to anthropomorphize, then to hate, the weather. I began to fantasize about building a time machine and going back to murder whoever invented wind. A dull ache from the constant pressure of pedaling possessed my right knee, which throbbed with each revolution of the cranks. Though my muscles were still strong, the discomfort in this joint limited the force I could put into each pedal stroke, slowing me down even further as I returned from the second lap. While I had been enjoying the all-expenses-paid tour of the desert, my father and Jen had somehow fabricated a giant motivational poster depicting a hand displaying a gang sign (a joke arising from an escape I'd once made from a Chicago gang that was hassling me). I wasn't feeling very good, and so, like an ambivalent movie critic, I was able to offer only a single unenthusiastic thumbs-up for their effort as I passed. I had no idea how I was going to manage the third circuit. I was gingerly turning the pedals, unable to apply enough force to take advantage of the downwind conditions. I knew coming back into town was going to be torturous in comparison, and I wasn't proven wrong. The wind had intensified to an insane level. Each time I looked at my current speed on my bike computer, I wished I had packed an antidepressant or two along with my salt tabs. I stared grimly at my bike odometer, watching the number creep ever so slowly from 94 to 95 to 96.

The wind ultimately played a role in a misfortune that would bring me to the low point of the day. I had reached the outskirts of town on the third loop and could see the first glimmers of light at the end of the tunnel. I was on track to finish the bike segment in about six hours, a more than acceptable time, considering the harsh conditions. I was coming to one of the final turns when I saw—I kid you not—a tumbleweed blowing toward me across the desert on an intersecting trajectory. This was a classic tumbleweed, straight out of a spaghetti western: about four feet in diameter and blowin' in the wind. Though it was moving quickly, it was still about two hundred yards away when I spotted it and seemed to pose little danger. I altered my course, but the tumbleweed matched the maneuver. It was now bearing down on me at a high rate of speed. Each time I zigged, it zagged, closing in on me like a guided missile. At contact, the tumbleweed sideswiped me like a linebacker engulfing a running back, partially entwining itself in the spokes of my back tire. Though it lacked the mass to knock me down directly, it caught me off balance, forcing me into a compensatory turn a little sharper than I'd planned. This move, combined with the hot asphalt and high tire pressure, was enough to cause a dramatic blowout of my rear tire. The tire's bare rim bit into the asphalt and I skidded down, scraping along the road before coming to rest on the shoulder. The tumbleweed left the scene, uninjured and without exchanging insurance information with me.

I picked myself up, concerned that I had broken something and would have to abandon the race. All my parts seemed to be intact, but I was bleeding from several places and my tire was now flat. The situation was so reminiscent of a stereotypical country and western moment that it was *almost* humorous. What wasn't funny was standing by the road and watching person after person I had struggled to pass now returning the favor. I needed to get back on the road quickly. Though I had never suffered a flat during a race, I possessed the know-how and the proper tools to fix the problem. I dumped out my toolkit and started working on changing the tire. I replaced the ruptured inner tube fairly easily, but ran into a problem putting the outer tire back on: my hands had absorbed so much road vibration that they were severely weakened, no longer strong enough to pop the tire back on the rim. After a stretch of bad luck, I finally caught a break: two volunteers from a nearby aid station spotted my predicament and came to my rescue. They replaced my tire on the rim. I inserted a portable $CO_2$ inflator and injected pressurized gas into the repaired tire. The tube held. I was back on the bike but had by then lost over twenty-five minutes on the side of the road.

Once I got back up to speed, it became apparent that something was still very wrong with the tire I had replaced. The bike was increasingly hard to handle, and it felt as though I were riding over speed bumps, even though the road was smooth. The crash may have done more damage to my bike than I realized. There was no other choice but to continue: I was fresh out of spare parts, so further repair was not an option. I was going as fast as I dared, still on the lookout in case the tumbleweed came back to finish the job, all the while praying that my machine would hold together for just a few more miles. By divine grace, it kept working long enough to deliver me to the finish line of the bike segment. Barely. Days later, at home after the race, I discovered that the replacement tube had popped again. Opening the tire, I saw that the inner tube had a huge kink in it (presumably the source of my bumpy ride), which had put enormous pressure on one segment of the tube. By all rights, it should have exploded again, forcing me to hoof it the last seven or eight miles. I took my miracles where I could. In the bike course finish chute, the volunteer who took my bike was shocked that I had completed the distance on a beginner-level bicycle. His exact words were, "A road bike? You gotta be shittin' me!" Feeling each and every yard I'd traveled, I was quite sure I was not shitting him.

Jen and my father, noting my overdue return, had moved over to the bike-to-run transition zone in time to see my stiff dismount and subsequent trudge into the changing tent. In half-Ironman races, I was used to quickly racking my bike and charging onto the run course within a matter of seconds. This time I sat down heavily on a bench and took a moment to recover my wits and take stock. The good news was that I was over 114 miles into the race. The bad news was that I felt like I was 114 miles into the race. Even so, I was far from winning the award for Worst-Looking Guy in the Changing Tent. People were haphazardly sprawled across chairs and on the ground, some of them dressing for the run, but many simply sitting and staring blankly into space. The scene bore a strong resemblance to an emergency room immediately after a major disaster. I wondered what the event's medical tent looked like.

I checked my cuts from the crash. The bleeding on my knee, shin, and elbow had been staunched, and everything seemed OK to run on. I pulled off my cycling cleats and slid my running shoes on with all the enthusiasm of a kid getting dressed for school. My bike helmet was replaced with a visor, and I pulled myself heavily to my feet, unconsciously letting a sigh ooze out of me. A volunteer came to take my bag. "You look good!" he said, with far more cheer than one should be allowed to use in such situations. "Think I'll go for a jog," I told him. "I'll be right back."

I had started getting in shape by running and, to achieve my Ironman goal, would have to finish the job by running. I'd run two stand-alone marathons previously, and after each one I'd wondered how I would feel if I had been softened up with a little swimming and biking first. I had now reached the point where I was qualified to answer this question: I felt like ten pounds of shit stuffed into a five-pound bag. Chief on my list of concerns was the sore knee I had nursed throughout the bike segment. Incredibly, it was now free of pain, and I had a full range of motion as I ran out of the transition zone and onto the run course. The crowds were again thick, and I fed off the excitement.

The run course was three circuits of a nine-mile loop. Though the course was pretty flat, there were some gentle slopes and a few legitimate climbs, especially significant for someone with tired legs. The previously bothersome wind was fast becoming my ally, helping me stay cool in the hot mid-afternoon conditions.

I had few expectations for the following miles. As an Ironman rookie, I couldn't rely on precedent to guess how far or how fast I could go. A preliminary answer was provided five minutes in, as it became crystal clear that running the entire distance without stopping was simply not going to happen. Although I was still under control at the moment, I could tell that I was exerting myself near the limits of my capacity. If I didn't change tactics, within an hour I would be taking a break (possibly in the hospital) whether I wanted to or not. The finish was many miles distant. I had to come up with a plan to get myself there. I would have to rely on my few remaining strengths to get through this. My innate talents formed a modest list: eating almost anything while exercising, thinking clearly and making adjustments during a competition, and setting aside my pride in order to do what needed to be done most efficiently. The first two abilities had already been tested extensively during the day, and I had largely succeeded in keeping my body energized and my exertions under control. Now it appeared that I would have to call on clear-eyed decision making and discipline to rein myself in and not overreach my capacities.

I had assumed I would begin to struggle late in the day and had developed a running plan for this eventuality. The idea was based on an experience from a previous marathon. In the late miles of the race, I had been trading positions with an older, fragile-looking guy. Like most everyone else in the race, I was running more or less constantly, but this fellow employed an unorthodox tactic: every mile, he would stop and walk for twenty or thirty seconds. Each time he did this, I would pass him, but then he would somehow catch up to me. It was an unusual strategy; typically, people who walk in races are exhausted and incapable of running further. Curious, I had begun experimenting with putting short walking breaks into my own training runs. I discovered that I was able to run much farther when I added these short breaks, with little loss in overall pace. Now seemed like an excellent time to try to stretch my endurance with this tactic. I decided to break the run into increments: five minutes of running followed by one minute of walking. To the untrained eye, it would appear as though I had unwisely spent too much of my energy on the bike or was quitting when things got hard. Indeed, more than a few people were already reduced to a walk at this early stage. In actuality, I was setting my ego aside to achieve a result. The objective was to get from point A to point B as quickly as possible, not to look good. By walking intermittently, I would stretch my energy reserves and increase my likelihood of doing more actual running overall.

For the first lap, all went according to plan. While running, I moved fluidly, passing person after person. During the minutes that I walked, those who continued running were able to gain perhaps twenty yards on me, only to be re-passed when I started running again. My cyclical schedule had the added benefit of breaking the large task into small, manageable bites. I saw my father and Jen at the beginning of the second lap and, for the first time of the day, got a very satisfying high-five from each of them. On the second lap, my passes became more frequent, as people who had run until they could run no more were reduced to the walking wounded. At one point, I actually stumbled into the head of the race. A mountain bike and a golf cart with a TV crew pulled alongside, and before I knew it, the female pro leader was running alongside me. The sheer excitement of being near the lead (not to mention the prospect of being on TV) was too much for even my tired legs to ignore, and I matched the leader's pace for a good five minutes. Finally I wished her luck and dropped back to a more sustainable speed.

My tactics, while solid, only delayed the inevitable. By the end of the second lap I was beginning to flag a bit. I compensated by shifting to four-minute running intervals, with one minute of walking in between. Later examination of my run splits indicated that my running speed never wavered, even toward the end. By remaining steady, I was moving forward while others faded. Still, the long, draining day was beginning to put me into something of an energy crisis. Running burns more calories per minute than biking, and it was impossible to completely absorb (and therefore replace) the energy I expended. At aid stations, I was making copious use of iced sponges and Gatorade before launching myself off in search of my next snack. Ten miles in, aid stations began offering defizzed cola to the racers. I'd never tried soda during a race, but I was feeling a strong desire for refined sugar, so I tried it. It was nothing short of a miracle drug, a boost that was huge in restoring both blood sugar and morale when I was so close to rock bottom. A few miles later, a new offering began to appear: lukewarm chicken broth, essentially a creative way to get salt back into the body. My need for both salt and sugar created an odd marriage of flavors. At each aid station I would take a cup of coke and a cup of broth, finding they mixed surprisingly well in my stomach. This was truly proof that I was able to eat anything, anytime.

At the end of the second lap, I saw my father and Jen, for what would likely be the last time before finishing. My watch and body indicated that it was time for a break, and I decided to use the opportunity to say hi and perhaps make a short speech expressing my gratitude for their support. As I pulled up, my father, understandably overstimulated by the comeback I was putting together, began peppering me with motivational nonsense. "Keep going! All go! No stop!" It seemed easier to start running again than to negotiate, and at that point, I was all about taking the path of least resistance. Without further ado, it was on to the third and final loop.

The details of the final circuit of the run course are a blurry haze of half-memories. I suspect a latent neural mechanism designed to limit the impact of mental trauma underlies this failure of memory. Months after the race, I heard a description of ultradistance triathlons that struck a chord: "All an Ironman really boils down to is running a half-marathon when you should be in the hospital." Who would want a vivid recollection of doing that? Only a few memories remain indelible. Daylight was fleeting, and the temperature was dropping rapidly as the sun settled into the desert horizon. I was past acute pain. Each step produced a deep reverberating ache that ran from my foot up to my groin and into my side. I was still passing people, more of them now than at any point before. The consequences of spending too much energy too early were never more apparent. At every aid station there were at least two or three people sitting on the curb, eyes glazed over and staring into space with an expression of fatigue and vague shame. As the day darkened into night, I crossed the bridge spanning Tempe Town Lake and headed down the final stretch.

Twice before I had seen the exit sign for the finish line, and twice before I had run past it to begin the next loop. This time there were no more laps to run. As I turned onto the finishing loop, the crowds realized another finisher was coming in, and broke into a spreading wall of enthusiastic applause. The intensity of the crowd's support for a stranger never ceases to be both touching and surprising; I must have looked as bad as I felt. I came around one more turn, and there was the finish line, lit up against the twilight. It was the first time I was 100 percent sure I was going to finish, and I dumped my remaining reserves into my legs, determined to finish in style. The finish-line announcer picked up on the action, bellowing the traditional announcement, "Noah Walton… you are an IRON-MAN!" as I crossed the finish line twelve hours and twenty-six minutes after starting.

Safe in the finish area, I had nowhere else to run. I ground to a complete halt for the first time all day. The sudden lack of motion was, for a moment, even more painful than the con-

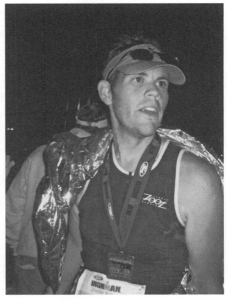

Immediately following the finish of Ironman Arizona. To use a friend's expression, "A cheeseburger is in order."

stant movement my legs had been rebelling against, so I started moving again. If I had stayed still, the blood vessels in my legs would have dilated ever so slightly and I would have fainted from a sudden lack of blood pressure. Someone gave me a Mylar blanket and a finisher's medal. In my finisher's photo, my suspicions about my appearance were confirmed: I resembled an ultra-fit vagrant. I grabbed another cup of flat cola (still couldn't get enough) and wandered out of the finishing area, dazed and confused. Fortunately, my father and Jen spotted and safely corralled me before I got too lost or started a fourth lap. They had already packed up my bike ("It smelled like an animal died on it") and now worked together to support my weight, forming an ungainly trio for the walk to the car. My body, at first so reluctant to let me stop moving, had enthusiastically embraced the reprieve, and I was having a hard time keeping up with my orderlies. Jen took the opportunity to shamelessly exploit the confluence of my weakened state, the large quantity of spandex I wore, and the Mylar emergency blanket I had fashioned into a crude cape. She whipped out her camera and began to film me, dubbing me the "metallic superhero." I was in no condition to prevent any catastrophes, including her posting this embarrassment on YouTube. I got a preview of just how sore I was going to be when I inadvertently stepped off the sidewalk and was unable to clear the five-inch curb to get myself back up there. I played it cool, pretending it was my decision to walk in the street next to the cars whizzing by.

From the backseat of the rental car, I cursed my aches as I struggled out of my crusty race duds and into a pair of jeans and a fresh shirt for the celebratory dinner at our traditional spot, the Cheesecake Factory. Getting out of the car required a bit of help from my dad, who pulled me to my feet like a dockworker hoisting a bag of grain. Upon standing, I was woozy to a degree that made exiting the swim (had it really only been earlier that morning?) seem like nothing. I promptly grayed out, and would have performed a spectacular face-plant into the parking lot if not for the timely intervention of my helpers, both of whom were earning their keep that day. Despite their diminutive stature, both my father and Jen are incredibly strong, and together, they manhandled me into the restaurant, probably not fully aware of how badly off I was. "You stink!" Jen informed me, in the same voice one might use to chastise a puppy. Of course, she *was* literally jammed into my armpit and supporting a significant fraction of my bodyweight. I didn't envy her the smell down there.

We got a table quickly. I believe the wait staff thought I was a very drunk celebrity with my entourage. Once I sat down and got some food into me, I began to feel better, and regaled my companions with the tales of the day. Despite big talk to the contrary, I was unable to finish my meal: chewing had become something of a chore. I tried a sip of my father's beer, which made me feel a little better and a lot drunker. Under guard again, I was escorted back to the car, and then the whole exercise was repeated to get me into the hotel when we arrived back there. I managed to take a shower, during which I confirmed that I was severely sunburned. With the pale skin that had been covered by clothing all day, the angry red sunburn on my exposed parts, and the darkening bruises from my crash, I was a walking punch line for the classic joke, "What's black and white and red all over?" After the shower, Jen gave me a leg massage. I got hungry again, and was eating a small sandwich and talking to Jen while she worked on what was left of my lower body. At one point, Jen asked me a question and I didn't answer. She looked up and saw that I had fallen asleep mid-conversation, sandwich still hanging out of my mouth. In her final act of race-day support, Jen tucked me in, removed the sandwich I was about to choke on … and proceeded to finish it herself.

# The Aftermath

*I've fallen, and I can't get up.*
—MRS. FLETCHER,
LIFE ALERT COMMERCIAL

Nine hours later, the act of rolling over triggered a cascade of aches and pains that was more than sufficient to wake me up bright and early. Getting around initially proved challenging. Some crawling was involved. Jen was still asleep amidst a pile of crumbs, so I crept to the lobby to see how I'd done in the race. My times were completely average for the swim and bike segments (the latter thanks to the flat tire), but I'd been buoyed by the strength of my finish. At the end of the day, when people were tired and hurting, I was at my best. In the last 26.2 miles, I had run past over a third of the competition, more than seven hundred people in all, and had moved myself into the top third of finishers. Later that morning, it was revealed that the race had the second-highest rate of people failing to finish in the history of Ironman triathlons, more than double the usual number. One in ten competitors had withdrawn or failed to finish within the seventeen-hour time limit, likely from the combination of heat and strong winds on the bike and run courses. Considering that, my finish was a pretty incredible way to celebrate my five-year anniversary of beginning to lose weight. Even after I'd become thin, it had taken a giant leap to reach this level of fitness and athletic achievement. It was my first Ironman, I had no lifelong athletic background, was the wrong size and shape for a triathlon, had the wrong equipment, and had never displayed any extraordinary athletic talents. It surprised me, even then, that the simple desire to do an Ironman and the willingness to approach the problem in a logical, stepwise fashion had carried me so far and allowed me to overcome a staggering array of reasons to fail.

The unofficial fourth leg of Ironman Arizona was the awards breakfast. Each time I moved, I felt like a hobbit was driving daggers into my legs. One guy cruised past, still wearing his competitor's wristband, going for a jog. I, on the other hand, had the stamina of a gorilla with one lung. I couldn't even stand very long without something (or somebody, as the song goes) to lean on. The most unusual type of soreness I had was located in my ribcage. A long day of breathing hard had fatigued the normally inexhaustible muscles of the lungs and diaphragm that support the expansion and contraction of the torso. This made it a little tiring just to sit around; I'd been up for three hours and already I needed a nap.

After the awards ceremony, Jen and I dropped my father off at the airport and went to get lunch. "What are you going to do now?" Jen asked.

"I don't know," I said. "Maybe I'll win it next year." I was joking, of course, but I felt a certain sense of possibility even as I spoke the words. The gap between myself at that time and the guy who'd won the race was a hell of a lot smaller than it had been five years, or even one year, previously. After the changes I'd gone through, how could I say anything was entirely out of the realm of possibility? It occurred to me, too, that there was no reason to limit myself to aiming for accomplishments solely in athletics. If I'd learned one thing, it was that I had within me the basic industry and drive to reach a high level in virtually anything I committed myself to completely. It was a very empowering realization.

After getting back to Chicago, I spent much of the next few months recovering. For the first week I simply lay on the couch, taking it easy and eating whatever I could get delivered. When I felt like getting up and about again, I gradually eased myself back into physical activity. I started gently; athletes are always at a high risk for injuries immediately after completing a race, and I wasn't planning anything else spectacular anytime soon after the Ironman. I needed some time to heal. Since reaching a reasonably high level of fitness, I had learned how to "borrow" from my body. In essence, I could push my performance past my known physical limits, but at a cost to be paid later. It's a lot like borrowing money from a lender; you get what you're looking for in the short term, but then you owe it back, with interest. In this case, my debt took the form of a feeling of deep fatigue, never immediately evident, but always lurking beneath the surface. Until that feeling went away, my body told me, I shouldn't start working hard again, lest there be consequences. I kept myself in good general condition, but left it at that.

Aside from my physical limitations, I seemed to have lost the mental drive to pursue my athletic development in the wake of the race. For the first time since losing weight, I had lost the impetus to get through (or even attempt) the demanding workouts required to reach and maintain a high level of fitness. Without the passion to work toward an ultimate goal, there was no point in putting myself through the motions. I was comfortable with the idea that I might have only one Ironman-type effort in me. I'd done what I'd set out to do. I'd demonstrated a level of fitness no one had thought me capable of. My experiment, at least in that regard, was a clear success. Though I enjoyed triathlons, I could live with the Arizona race being the last of my career.

I suspected that my lack of motivation was closely linked to my physical lethargy; my mind and body were working in synergy to remain inactive long enough to repair and rebuild. Whatever the case, there was little to do but wait until I was ready to go again. If, or when, my body was ready to let me do another race, it would let me know. The extreme level of fitness I had reached wasn't the norm, nor was it easy to maintain, and I had developed to the point where I was able to stay in good enough shape without a particular goal aside from general fitness. Nor was my identity at stake; I didn't define myself by athletics, and I would always be able to find some other pursuit to satisfy me if need be.

My self-imposed retirement lasted about three months, roughly as long as a bear hibernates. All of a sudden, I began feeling more like my old self and was ready to pick up where I'd left off. In Florida, I would have been out of luck; the summer months were a dead zone on race calendars there on account of the soaring temperatures and stifling humidity. In the Midwest, the opposite was true; summer and fall were the only times you could hold an event and not run the risk of waking up to six inches of snow on race day. There were opportunities to be had, but only if I acted quickly to prepare.

With all due caution, I began to cycle up, increasing the length of my longer workouts and focusing on proper diet. Unlike the raw, blustery days of early spring, the fine summer weather had brought out the crowds to keep me company. The lakefront path was teeming with all manner of sun worshippers and outdoor enthusiasts. This posed some problems. Though the company provided a welcome sightseeing diversion while I ran, it was nothing short of suicidal to try biking with any speed on a weekend. Children, in particular, were unpredictable human missiles, prone to zipping directly into my path at any moment. People at the opposite end of the size spectrum were just as dangerous. Though not fleet of foot, fat people who traveled the path were often too discombobulated or lazy or simply physically unable to turn their heads to spot approaching cyclists as they waddled along the path. These human roadblocks were well known to the University of Chicago's Velo Club, with which I had, on occasion, taken to riding. When riding in a group, we would call out their presence as a warning to the rest of the group, just as we would a car or pothole. There was even a slang term for them: DFPs—Disoriented Fat People. Usually, DFPs were at least predictable in their habitat, roaming in loose packs around touristy establishments and the occasional food kiosk.

As the weather turned warm, Chicago offered me another training opportunity that I experienced all too infrequently: open water swimming. Lake Michigan was finally getting warm enough to swim in. It was surprising to hear that, in spite of its proximity to the city, the lake's water quality was generally regarded as being very safe for swimming. It was also free from predators; in comparison to Florida's waterways, remarkably few alligators live in the waters of Lake Michigan. On the other hand, despite the assurances I had received that the lake would grow warm enough to sustain human life, I had not yet seen any Chicagoans in the lake as April gave way to May. The few times I had grown bold enough to dip my toe in, it was pretty damn cold. Still, the prospect of getting out of the pool and into open water was too appealing to resist for very long. On Memorial Day weekend, the official start of outdoor swimming at city beaches, I grabbed my wetsuit and headed out to the lake.

Even on a perfect day in late May, the 57th Street beach was almost completely deserted, save for a couple of bored sweater-clad lifeguards and a ragged-looking bum in no condition for anything more ambitious than sunbathing and drinking Boone's Farm. The complete lack of people gave me an inkling that this might not be my finest idea ever. I hadn't seen any ice floating in the lake in over a month, but I wasn't taking any chances—I would not become the butt of a joke about the Ironman who didn't float. I put on my wetsuit and two swim caps and said a prayer to the patron saint of the circulatory system as I waded in. Though the wetsuit protected my torso and legs, everything else was instantly chilled, and this southerner learned a valuable lesson: water temperatures in the fifties are MUCH colder than the corresponding air temperature. The deeper the water, the colder it got, as the sun's rays failed to penetrate the murky depths of the lake. It felt like I was swimming through a submerged meat locker. The beach was located in a shallow man-made harbor, with a line of buoys about three hundred yards offshore providing a demarcation for boat traffic. My immediate plan was to swim the length of the buoy line and back, about a mile or so. Spotting the leftmost buoy, I made for it with all due haste, my core body temperature falling fast.

My plan hit a snag almost immediately. Within the city limits of Chicago, it is apparently illegal to swim off of a beach past where the water becomes chest-deep. By heading out to deeper water, I triggered the response of the city's beach rescue system. At the very mention of this, many of you may now be picturing a Midwestern version of Pamela Anderson perkily bouncing along on a jet ski and executing a flawless dive to pull this hapless swimmer from the dank clutches of the lake. I would have been fine with that, but it didn't quite go down that way. I had been making good progress when I was rudely poked in the back by a pole of some sort. Peering upwards, I saw that the pole was actually an oar belonging to a dirty rowboat piloted by a skeletal septuagenarian. He reminded me less of *Baywatch* and more of the fabled boatman of Greek mythology, there to escort me across the River Styx and into the underworld. This boatman was angry, possibly because I had seemed to decline his services in favor of swimming directly into the afterlife. From his irritable diatribe, I gathered I was to reverse course immediately.

Returning to terra firma under my own power, I was informed of the regulations against swimming in the lake, which put a significant kink in my plans. Seeking clarification, I braved the beach's bureaucracy. I found my geriatric rescuer's land-based supervisor, a 300-plus-pound woman (who would have served as an excellent flotation device) and pleaded my case. Eventually, I found a loophole in the rules: though it was illegal to swim in deep water off the *beach*, it was acceptable to swim as far as I liked off of the adjacent rocky shoreline. Essentially, the regulations were in place because there would be significantly more paperwork to fill out were I to meet my maker on the lifeguards' watch. It's good to know that people care about you.

One week later, attempt *deux* at lake swimming was uninterrupted and deeply fulfilling. The simple pleasure of swimming in one direction for more than twenty-five yards without having to turn around was invigorating. The next weekend I returned for another outing. I laboriously picked my way through the rocks and had a nice, if chilly, dip. Forty-five minutes later I waded ashore and peeled off my wetsuit, ready to get dressed and go home. There was one problem: I couldn't find my clothes. It was a calm day; there was no way they could have been blown or washed away, so I was left with the conclusion that someone had stolen them while I swam. I had been warned about the crime in Chicago, especially on this beach, which was a little seedier than those bordering the ritzy uptown neighborhoods. But still—what kind of person sees pawnable value in used clothes and a pair of flip-flops?

My anger began to mount. *What kind of scumbag crackhead would steal used clothes?* It wasn't as though my stuff had been sitting there all day or was obviously abandoned. Cursing everyone who passed as a potential thief, I made one final reconnaissance of the area and began the barefoot half-mile walk to my apartment, wetsuit slung over my shoulder, wearing only a Speedo and a foul expression. I was sure the tourists in front of the nearby Museum of Science and Industry would really appreciate the fashion statement I was making. I had reached the entrance to the pedestrian tunnel under Lake Shore Drive when a woman yelled after me to stop. She asked me if I was missing some clothes. Thinking that perhaps she was the one who had stolen them and was now stricken with guilt at the sight of me, I fixed her with my steeliest gaze and asked her if she thought people normally strutted around like this. The shame, it seemed, was to be mine. She had volunteered to lead a group of inner-city kids on a cleanup of the lakefront area. One of the youngest kids had mistaken my neatly folded clothing for common detritus and had innocently carried it off. As she explained the situation, two of the older kids fished my clothes out of a trash bag and returned them to me. Foot firmly wedged in mouth, I sheepishly thanked the counselor and her volunteers for their well-meaning work. I put on my clothes, which now had the warm yeasty smell of beer. To date, this is the closest I have come to encountering Chicago's fabled syndicate of beach thieves.

My training was once again going well and I was feeling really good, so I began making plans for upcoming events. The U.S. National Triathlon Championships, for which I had qualified the previous year in Miami, were to be held in Innsbrook, Missouri, just outside of St. Louis. This happened to be within driving distance of Chicago, and an opportunity to participate in an actual national championship was far too enticing to pass up. Since this was a chance to test myself at the highest level of amateur competition, I devoted myself to physically peaking for the race. With the championships scheduled for mid-September, I registered for an event a month earlier, to use as a tune-up. After having geared my training toward the Ironman for so long, and then taking several months off from racing, I figured it would be good to get re-accustomed to the different speed of the "short distance" races.

My tune-up event was the Whirlpool Steelhead 70.3, one of the largest triathlons in the country, held in southwest Michigan. Steelhead was almost a hometown event for those living in Chicago, and a special check-in for the race was held downtown the weekend before the race. This allowed city dwellers to collect their registration materials and drive to the race site the morning of the event, sparing them the need for lengthy round-trips. This pre-registration was something of a logistical necessity, as the event was held in Benton Harbor, Michigan, a beautiful but tiny hamlet that lacked sufficient hotel rooms for the race's 2,400 registered participants. Though my race preparations were usually meticulous, thinking of Steelhead as a mere tune-up had made me inattentive; I completely forgot about the local check-in for the race. This put me in a difficult situation: I could either drive two hours to Benton Harbor the day before the race to register and rack my bike, drive two hours back to Chicago, and then drive out again on race morning, or I could try to find a hotel in the Benton Harbor area. The latter was clearly not going to happen. Every nearby hotel room had been snapped up long ago by people with more prescience than I. Strike one.

Ultimately, I came up with a solution that would simultaneously save me money and free me from making multiple round trips. Race head-quarters were supposedly on the beach of southeastern Lake Michigan. If I brought a sleeping bag, I could spend the night before the race sleeping there, under the stars. The weather forecast was favorable, and with this plan I wouldn't have the stress of fighting traffic on race morning. The more I thought about it, the more confident I became that this was the best idea I'd had in a long time.

The race was on a Saturday. I arrived and checked in on Friday afternoon, attended the pre-race dinner, and then struck out in search of supplies. I had suffered my second slip in attention before leaving Chicago, neglecting to purchase the special energy bars and drinks I usually consumed during these kinds of events. Usually something very similar can be found at a grocery store…only I couldn't find the grocery store in Benton Harbor. After driving around for an hour and wasting much emotional and physical energy, I finally settled on the only food-selling store I could find: a Walgreen's drugstore. Ever tried to get specialized food at a Walgreen's? I don't recommend it. I did manage to pick up some Gatorade, but the only energy snacks I could find were super-sugary trail mix bars. My nutritious pre-race meal? Sea salt bagel crisps. Strike two, with a vengeance.

The race staging area was almost deserted by the time I returned to the park at dusk. I dragged my sleeping bag out to the beach and enjoyed the spectacular sight of the sun sinking into Lake Michigan while eating a bag of M&Ms. I felt at peace with the world. Once the stars came out I set my alarm clock for 6 AM, a comfortable ninety minutes before the race was scheduled to start, congratulated myself on my brilliant plan, then curled up in my sleeping bag and drifted off to the gentle lapping of waves.

The next morning I was stirred to wakefulness not by the sound of my alarm, but by a couple of people walking by me. They were both wearing wetsuits and were walking in the direction of the swim start. It seemed early for that … unless my alarm hadn't gone off! In a state of panic, I seized my alarm clock. *Whew.* There were still five minutes until it was set to go off. Crisis averted! Just to be safe, I checked my cell phone's clock as well. According to my phone, it was almost 7:00, a full hour later than I thought. Crisis restored! Despite being only a short drive from Chicago, Benton Harbor is in the Eastern Time Zone, and I had forgotten about the time change. My cell phone, which received a continually updated digital signal, was telling the truth: I was *really* late. My third strike, and the race hadn't even started yet. With only thirty minutes to get ready and get to the start, I was riding a rollercoaster of panic. To complicate matters further, the swim course for the Steelhead ran point-to-point, rather than in a loop, and it started over a mile up the beach. My time frame for getting to the start went from tight to almost impossible. After a wild, haphazard scramble to clothe myself and prepare my gear, I found myself running down the beach and trying to put on my wetsuit at the same time. I arrived, out of breath and sweating, with about 60 seconds to spare.

*At least I got a warm-up in,* I thought, as I joined the crowd on the starting line. I had literally seconds to come up with a plan for handling the swim course. The path we were to swim was marked by a line of buoys running parallel to the beach, some 200 yards offshore. The only rule was that we keep the buoys on our right. The first buoy was significantly down the shore from where we started, and the most direct route to it went at a 45-degree entry angle from the beach. With my brain in overdrive, I noticed that if I were to run down the beach until I was even with the first buoy and then swim directly toward it, I wouldn't have to swim as far. It looked like a legal possibility. Using my seventh-grade geometry skills, I knew that this made for a longer distance overall, but more than half of it would be covered by relatively fast-paced running and wading through the shallow part of the lake. Before I could carefully weigh the pros and cons of the plan, the gun for the race went off. Sometimes during a race, there's a little voice in my head that advises me. Right now, the little voice was saying, *C'mon Noahmeister! Man up, try the shortcut.* For lack of a better idea, I complied. As I suspected, pretty much everyone went directly at the first buoy, heading into the lake while I ran down the shoreline. I zipped along the packed wet sand of the beach, almost colliding with a surprised spectator but nonetheless surging ahead of the main field. As I drew even with the first buoy, I made a hard left, directly into Lake Michigan. There are few advantages to being tall, usually limited to seeing over crowds and changing light bulbs. I now discovered another: I was able to wade a surprisingly long way into the lake, using a rather dainty high-stepping technique, before I had to start swimming. The race director spotted my legal shortcut tactic. "Look at the tall guy go!" he bellowed into the microphone. As I was also very interested in how the tall guy was doing, I looked left to see where I was in relation to the competition. The "Walton Maneuver" had paid off handsomely: everyone else was mired in a pack of thrashing swimmers, and my gambit had opened up a lead on the field of almost a hundred yards.

A final dive took me into to the murky water. Three minutes after nearly missing the start of the race, I was now leading it. I promptly experienced my first ever full-blown delusion of grandeur. An internal dialogue played out in my head that went a little something like this:

> *Optimism:* Holy shit, Noah! You're leading the race. You're a stud!
> *Pessimism:* Easy on the trash talk, pal. Last time I checked, you were a lousy swimmer.
> *O:* Shut up and swim faster! You're going to lead this thing start to finish!
> *P:* I wouldn't get too comfortable being in front.

Before the two voices came to blows, the issue of my impending triumph was settled when a former collegiate swimmer came flying by as though I wasn't even moving. And he had company. While my dreams of winning were crushed like a ripe grape in a wine press, I had at least tasted that grape, however briefly, and it was sweet.

The rest of the day went pretty well. For one of the first times in a race, I didn't work as hard as I probably could have; it was my first race in a while and I didn't want to put myself out of commission for a long time afterward by pushing past my limits. One of the first things I had done after Ironman Arizona was to dole out the cash for a nice new triathlon bike. It was bright yellow and black, and I dubbed it El Abejorro ("The Bumblebee," a nickname I had picked up in soccer for my tenacity and remarkable lack of speed). With better equipment, I set a new personal best on the rolling bike course and was feeling great when I started the run. The course was a lollypop-shaped affair that took two loops of the Whirlpool corporate campus—a particularly humane design, considering that it meant we didn't have to run past the finish line on the way to the second loop. Even though I took it easy, I set a new personal best for the run by a full five minutes. Overall, I also set a new personal best for the half-Ironman distance and even came heartbreakingly close to winning some hardware by placing fourth in my division. It was as good as I could have expected for a warm-up event. More importantly, I now felt the fire for racing that had been missing for the past few months. It was good to be back, and I felt I might be on the cusp of breaking through to the next level. And in a month, I would get my chance to do just that.

# National Championships

The Steelhead 70.3 had been a mere appetizer for the U.S. National Championships six weeks later. I had done everything possible to give this race my best effort. At Steelhead I'd guarded against exhausting, injuring, or otherwise burning myself out, and had since been diligently getting ready for the upcoming challenge. I'd taken a methodical approach to my preparations, leaving no stone unturned in searching for an advantage. I'd researched the topography of the Nationals race course and discovered that hills were the order of the day. To adapt myself to such terrain, I took two trips to Madison, Wisconsin to train on the hilly route of the Ironman course there. I even pre-bought my race snacks and booked an honest-to-god hotel room near the race site in advance.

A race on the national stage was another opportunity to step up to the next level in my development. Throughout the whole of the journey I had been on, I had been driven by personal motivations and had set my own goals and expectations. Initially, by necessity, these motivations were to accomplish goals that were small or relatively unimpressive to most people, things like running a mile or starting a weight loss program. As I strung small successes together, the goals became bigger. Run a 5K. Finish a 15K. These were somewhat impressive to an average, sedentary person, but still quite pedestrian to anyone of even modest athletic ability. As I improved at this intermediate level, I expanded the scope of the new challenges I adopted. Bike the length of Florida. Finish an Ironman. Tests of this sort are considered significant measures of intestinal fortitude by even accomplished athletes (and often as acts of utter lunacy by the average person). By finishing an Ironman, I had more or less run out of mountains to climb, in terms of finding bigger, tougher races. The next phase of my development seemed to be in improving the quality of my finishes. I had won a few awards for finishing in the top three in several local races, but had never managed to place at a major race until my surprise second-place finish at Miamiman, which had also been my ticket to Nationals. Since qualifying, I'd drawn achingly close to high finishes, and I thought I was due for a breakthrough. This race, however, would be a difficult place to make the jump. The U.S. National Championships field was primarily comprised of competitors who had qualified to be there. My performance against this stiff competition would be an excellent indicator of how I compared to the top individuals in the sport. Was I going to do well? I tended to doubt it, but I didn't really know. As they say, that's why they run the race.

I drove to St. Louis the day before the race. The venue was more beautiful than any I had ever seen before. The swim was held in the glassy lake of the Innsbrook Resort and the course was well marked. The bike course was set to follow local roads with little vehicular traffic, and the run course threaded through shady deciduous forest on hard-packed gravel trails. The rumors about hills had been true. The only flat part of the course was the swim. Especially within the resort property, there were some dismayingly steep slopes that would be difficult to navigate on a triathlon bike. I could only assume that someone had thought the top athletes would appreciate the additional challenge.

Nationals marked only the second time (the first being the previous month's race in Michigan) that I was attempting a long triathlon without a support person in tow. I had become accustomed to traveling by myself but had never grown terribly fond of it. In particular, I harbored a special distaste for eating alone—a person sitting alone in a restaurant is one of the most depressing sights I can imagine. As I checked in to my hotel, I inquired as to the presence in town of quality purveyors of prepared foodstuffs. The clerk (completely barefoot and still with one eye on a Bollywood soap opera) recommended Applebee's with a straight face. If there's one thing I hate more than eating alone, it's eating alone at a soulless mid-range corporate chain restaurant. In the restaurant, I sat at the bar and listened to two locals locked in debate over who would prevail in a boxing match between Jesus and Santa Claus. I vowed never to travel solo again. Back at the hotel, I gave my dad a call. I told him I felt good, and that I thought I might have a good race in me the next day.

A freakish cold snap for September plunged temperatures into the thirties overnight. The morning air was chilly, and frost covered my car. I had packed lightly—too lightly—for the trip and was wearing every scrap of clothing I had brought as I prepared to head to the resort. If there was an upside to my shivering, it was that conditions would be favorably cool as the day wore on, helping me conserve energy otherwise spent on dissipating waste heat. This was of no consolation as I set up my bike to the sound of chattering teeth and the sight of billowing crystalline clouds of breath. With due haste, I set up my gear and warmed up with a power-walk back to the car. My options for keeping warm were limited, so I decided to make a bold fashion statement by putting on my wetsuit for warmth. For the next fifteen minutes, I pretended that neoprene was the new black this season. Finally, I headed down to the beach for the swim start. "Heading down" is a particularly apt term, considering the terrain; Innsbrook Lake sat in a bowl some seventy feet below the transition zone. In that sense, not even the swim course was flat.

Competing in the championship were three hundred qualifying athletes, divided into three starting groups. Before the start, seventy-seven-year-old Sister Madonna Buder, the oldest woman to have completed an Ironman (and, of course, also a competitor in this event) said a few words, and the national anthem was played. Then it was go time. I was in the third group with the rest of the Clydesdale division, the big guys I would be competing against. The first two groups were sent on their way, and it was evident that some really strong swimmers had come to visit northeast Missouri. Daniel Bretscher, the eventual champion, opened up a big lead during the swim, and was almost out of the water by the time my group was called to the beach. I jumped into the lake to get a few strokes in and loosen up my shoulders. The water was much warmer than the air temperature, which still hovered in the upper thirties, and I lounged in its comparative warmth as long as I could. Badgered by the race director, I slowly made my way back to the beach to join the hundred or so athletes crowding at the water's edge. Once out of the water, I was freezing again, this time with the added benefit of being wet. For the first (and perhaps only) time in my life, I was really looking forward to starting a swim. "Anyone want to spoon me until the gun goes off?" I asked the assembled crowd. There were more than a few takers, but before the scenario could be enacted, the cannon went off and my national championships were underway.

I had made a deal with myself during the drive down. There was no guarantee I would ever be able to qualify to get back here again. This might be my only chance to compete at this level. Since I had earned the opportunity, I was going to use it as I saw fit. In that spirit, I vowed to be aggressive from the beginning. In previous races, the swim had been an ordeal to be survived, used as a warm-up for my legs, which were stronger at biking and running. Today, I was looking to keep myself in contact with swimmers who were much faster than I normally was. I was going to have to use every trick I had accumulated over the past two years and, like the pros at Ironman Arizona, stay focused all day long.

With increasing experience, I had found the swim in triathlons to be surprisingly strategic. The better, faster swimmers were always eager to shed slower swimmers who sought the draft from their feet. To do this, the more powerful swimmers often began races at a near-sprint before settling into a more comfortable level of effort. In order to stay with the faster swimmers so that they would pull me along, I would also have to sprint at the start. I gambled that the early expenditure of energy would be worth it. Straight away, I established a good position and found a fast pair of feet to hang onto. As we settled into a rhythm, I managed to get a sense of my position through stolen glances between strokes. I was realistic: I had zero chance of winning the open race. My body was too big to ever be really competitive in that regard. However, if I played my cards just right, I might be able to manage a good finish relative to the other big men in my division. All competitors wore color-coded swim caps, and it was easy to track the bright orange caps attached to big swimming bodies. Of the competitors in my cohort, one of them— probably a high school or collegiate swimmer—was rapidly pulling away from the pack. I hoped he wasn't too strong a biker or runner. Two others had a healthy lead on me, and another fellow was just a few yards ahead. I established my pace to match this last fellow, keeping him as close as possible. It was working; halfway through I was still in contact with him. On the return to the beach, my shoulders began to ache from the effort of keeping up, and I lost focus briefly. Though it was only a second or two, this lapse in concentration was all it took for a gap to open up between the swimmer I was following and myself. Without the benefit of a draft, I quickly fell back, and had lost another hundred yards on fourth place by the finish of the swim. Though I had succeeded in keeping reasonably close, I was furious over my lapse in concentration. I was determined to make up time in the first transition.

Almost as an afterthought, I checked my watch as I came out of the water. Thirty-one minutes and change, my fastest swim by a wide margin. I crossed the beach and charged up the first steep hill of the day, pumping my arms against the slope. I transitioned quickly, jumped on my new bike, and was on the bike course without a moment wasted. The course for the ride consisted of two identical twenty-eight-mile loops that threaded through the Innsbrook Resort before venturing into the neighboring country roads. Finding a comfort zone early on the bike was particularly difficult today. My heart rate was soaring after I scaled the small mountain connecting the beach and the transition zone, and the savagely steep hills of the resort gave no quarter for cardiovascular recovery. I was spending energy, too much and too early, but my efforts had yielded a dividend: I had made up the time difference in swim time with my nearest competitor and passed him to move into fourth place within my division. So far, so good.

As I left the resort, the terrain leveled out and I finally found a good rhythm. I was mentally focused and turning the pedals at a good, high cadence. The course wasn't giving much away today. Missouri offered an inexhaustible array of rolling hills, and the only flat section was set directly into the prevailing wind. Normally, the bike segment is where I began to make my move up in the field. I would begin to reel in the fast swimmers from previous groups almost immediately and would generally continue to do so through the entirety of the bike course.

The biggest difference between a national championship and a regular event was that here everyone was a strong swimmer *and* a strong biker. Even though I was riding well, I passed very few athletes, most of them women from the previous wave. It was a real testament to the quality of the field. I was certainly more than holding my own, though; few people passed me, and I did manage to pull a few people back in myself. One of them was the third-place competitor in my division, whom I passed on one of the umpteen climbs of the course. I was now looking to be on the podium, if I could maintain my position. While I still had forty miles to go, the thought of being remotely in contention to place was a wondrous drug, and I turned the cranks even faster, trying to put as much real estate between myself and those now chasing me. I was almost too enthusiastic; shortly after the halfway point, I was navigating another of the steep hills of the resort and applied so much torque while shifting that my bike chain fell off. It was a simple fix, but it cost me two precious minutes to replace the chain and get moving. I was still in third, but I had certainly lost some of the cushion between myself and anyone who could run. "What did I ever do to you?" I yelled at my bike as I hopped back on.

The second loop flew by. I was so focused that I was barely aware of the passage of time. I was pushing even harder now, and I maintained an even pace on each lap of the bike course, despite the brief pit stop on the second circuit. Considering the hills, it was my best ride ever. More important, I was getting stronger as the race wore on. At the bike-to-run transition, I performed a flawless flying dismount from my bike and tore through with one of the fastest transition times of the day. Someone saw the "C" (for Clydesdale division) written on my calf and yelled out that I was eight minutes behind the leaders.

My position was far from guaranteed. A strong run on a difficult, sloping course would be necessary just to fend off the charge of those behind me. The same run could move me past those who had spent their energy unwisely. Eight minutes was a lot to make up over only thirteen miles, especially in a race like this, where I would have to run a full forty seconds per mile faster than my competition just to get close at the finish. Still, trying to do so was the best way to guarantee I would stay in third position, or even…you never know.

We would be running two identical laps through some very hilly paths, part gravel, and part pavement. Since the morning, temperatures had risen to very comfortable levels, and it was still far from hot. That would give me an essential boost, as the course routing turned out to be the most punishing I had ever run on. The course began with a short uphill section, followed by almost a mile of winding descents that I would have to climb before the finish of each of the two laps. As odd as it sounds, running downhill is just as hard on the legs as going uphill. When descending a slope, you tend to take large steps to stay balanced, transferring tremendous impact forces that the legs and spine must bear. The unusual muscular contractions that absorb the shock wear out your legs and hips surprisingly quickly, especially if you're not petite. Climbing stairs the next day would be inadvisable.

From my vantage point as a chaser, the course was ideal for monitoring a time deficit. There were four out-and-back sections on each lap, offering me the opportunity to keep an eye on those in front of and behind me. Midway through the first lap, I caught a glimpse of both of the leaders in my division. They were easy to spot—two guys who towered over smaller competitors, running together and still almost a full mile ahead of me. The mere sight of the competition was enough to give me another little bit of motivation. Other than my time deficit, things were shaping up well. Running in a triathlon is all about finding a rhythm; you're already achy and a little stiff from having stayed in the aerodynamic position on the bike for so long, and you just want to get your legs into a pattern to carry you along. The course was well-marked for distances, and I was getting rough mile splits off my watch. In spite of the uneven course, I was running far faster than ever before, on track for a personal best. Better yet, no one was threatening to catch me from behind.

At the halfway point I saw the leaders again. One of them had opened up a sizable advantage on the other and looked to be pulling away. He ignored me as he went past; perhaps I was too far back to constitute a threat. I probably was; a check of my watch showed me still six minutes behind, having made up only two minutes during the first half of the run. But the second-place guy was only four minutes in front of me, and he seemed to be struggling. As we passed each other going in opposite directions, his eyes flickered over to me, and I saw worry in them. If I hurried, I thought I might be able to catch him for second place.

With four miles left in the race, I caught my first glimpse of the back of his jersey. He was clearly in distress now, leaning slightly to the right and limping from the effect of the hills. I felt as though an invisible rubber band was pulling us together as my legs slowly, inexorably closed the distance. I drew alongside and passed him with no response. I had just moved into second place at the U.S. National Championships. That seemed to be the best I could do; six minutes back with four miles to go was too much to make up. Or was it? On the very next out-and-back segment, I spotted the leader. I had expected him to still be far in front, but I had gained ground quickly. He was only about four minutes in front of me, and he wasn't looking so fresh anymore.

It was time to make a quick decision. The guy I had passed for second was quickly falling back, and no one else was threatening to close in on me. I could probably protect my position and cruise home without doing too much damage. Second place would be a fine result. *Or you could try to catch him and win it*, a voice in me whispered. Never, in a million years, did I think I would be so close to first place this late in the race, even with everything I'd done in the previous months and years to reach this point. Now that I was there, what was I going to do with it? What was I going to let limit me? After years of dieting and exercising, all I knew was to go at things hard. I focused on turning my legs over just a little faster, keeping my stride relaxed and fluid. The same thoughts ran through my head: *Just keep doing what you're doing. Don't fade. Just stay strong.*

With two-and-a-half miles to go, we hit the final out-and-back section. I was only two minutes behind now. The first place runner definitely saw me this time. Now it was my turn to ignore him; I looked straight ahead, trying to appear strong while covertly sizing him up from behind the dark lenses of my sunglasses. He looked more than mildly concerned about the rate at which I was closing in. One and a half miles to go. I caught sight of him again. I drew closer; I could see the sweat-streaked "C" on his calf. Everyone else who mattered was gone; it was down to the two of us. The first place guy had joined two other runners. At the last aid station, I caught the group. I pulled out my old trick from the Miamiman, feigning a stop and then trying to covertly zip past amidst the flurry of cups and iced sponges. But there would be no sneak attacks today. My competitor caught me red-handed in the pass and responded to the move, matching me stride for stride. Now we were running together, less than a mile from the finish.

The effort to catch up had left me spent. The road was swimming in and out of focus. Lines of salt had formed on my face and clothes, and my teeth were exposed in a perpetual grimace of pain. My goals at this point were figuring out how to drop this guy and not dropping dead from hypoxia. In that order. We covered the last flat section of the course, still step for step. I didn't need to look to know this—I could hear his footsteps and breathing over the pounding of my own heart. I felt twinges of cramps; I had stopped drinking fluids long ago, and I was starting to suffer from dehydration. None of that mattered now. This was one on one to the finish.

Three-quarters of a mile left. I had to make a move before the end. There was no way I could win a sprint finish on my failing legs. The last climb—a cruel, twisting half mile—loomed in front of us. That would have to be where I did it. It was now or never.

I had started this whole experiment to see if I could create something out of essentially nothing—an elite athlete out of a completely sedentary, obese person. Now, I needed to make something happen once again, and I had nothing left to do it with. How could I somehow push my body to win this one last victory? In the past five years, I'd bottled up many unpleasant memories of my life as a fat person: taunting in school, the expressions of revulsion on girls' faces at my appearance, humiliations in gym class. The scraps I had kept of all these negative images became a sort of kindling for an internal fire. I took the frustration, rage, and disappointment I had experienced, and I asked myself, *What are you going to do about it now?* I felt a spark.

We hit the climb. I maintained my pace for a moment, listening to the breathing of the man beside me. As his breathing deepened and took on the thin raspiness of a gasp, I hit him with the biggest surge I could muster. For a second, five seconds, he stayed with me. *If this hurts me, it's killing him,* I told myself. I didn't look to find out if I was right. I didn't have to. The breathing on my shoulder grew fainter. The footsteps faded. I didn't look back. It was either enough or it wasn't.

I reached the top of the climb, free of my pursuer and with an answer to the question I had investigated for so long. In high school, I'd needed to be measured for an extra-extra-extra large uniform for marching band. Five years prior, I couldn't run around a football field. Today, I crossed the finish line at the national triathlon championships, in first place in my division and a long way from where I'd started.

# MUSINGS ON WEIGHT LOSS

# Studying Weight Loss

*The successful person has the habit of doing
things failures don't like to do. They don't
like doing them either necessarily. But their
dislike is subordinated to the strength of
their purpose.*

—E.M. GRAY

During the course of my own fitness experiment, I became interested
in learning what scientists who studied obesity were learning, so as to
place my findings within the context of those of the larger scientific
community. With their large-scale clinical studies, reams of statistics,
and objectivity, perhaps others would notice something I had missed.

The idea of studying what works in weight loss is hardly novel. In the
United States, one of the best resources for studying the phenomenon
is the National Weight Control Registry (NWCR),[15] which tracks individuals who have lost a minimum of thirty pounds and kept it off for at
least one year.[16] By studying these individuals and comparing them to
their less successful counterparts, researchers hope to identify the behaviors, attitudes, and other factors that contribute positively to weight
loss.

Many of the studies conducted on individuals in the NWCR echoed
and reinforced my major conclusions. Surprisingly, there seem to be
very few consensus patterns among successful dieters. NWCR mem-

bers used a wide variety of methods for losing weight; they are randomly divided among common dietary strategies such as restricting certain foods, limiting portions, and counting calories. Half of the participants used professional help (i.e., a physician, dietician, or commercial weight-loss program) and the other half worked independently. Sometimes a triggering event (such as suffering a heart attack, reaching an all-time high weight, or seeing themselves in a mirror) prompted weight loss, but often no such event existed.

There are only a few behaviors conserved in (i.e., common among) those who successfully lose weight. One of them is combining diet and exercise. Eighty-nine percent of successful dieters reported using both diet and exercise to control their weight, with only 10 percent using diet alone and only 1 percent using exercise alone. A high volume of exercise was another predictor for weight loss; successful dieters reported an average of one hour of moderate-to-brisk activity a day. Another factor for success was eating breakfast every day: a bare 4 percent of successful dieters reported never eating breakfast. Although this predictor is somewhat nonintuitive, it matches my personal experience perfectly. While fat, I rarely ate breakfast. There was never time in the morning, and I wasn't hungry. As I viewed things then, any time I didn't feel compelled to eat, I probably shouldn't. After beginning the regimen of intermittent fasting (and later, exercising), I would awake ravenously hungry on days when I could eat, promptly rushing to the refrigerator. This was a habit I adopted full-time after losing weight. In all, I found that I had independently adopted virtually all of the major consensus behaviors for successful weight loss that this large-scale study identified.

This confluence of findings wasn't terribly surprising. The efficacy of diet and exercise is so well established that it's almost become dogmatic. Multiple branches of the government (including the Departments of Health and Human Services and Agriculture and the Centers for Disease Control and Prevention) issue national standards for exercise and

diet that incorporate portions of the above-mentioned scientific findings. For example, the new "food pyramid," which promotes both portion control and the restriction of certain food types, was introduced in
2005 to replace the then twelve-year-old "four food groups" paradigm.
Recently introduced guidelines on exercise have expanded to advocate
an average of sixty minutes of moderate-to-brisk exercise per day, closely paralleling the amount of activity reported by NWCR respondents.

From my unique perspective on losing weight, I was able to add to
the list an admittedly less quantifiable behavior leading to successful
weight loss: persistence. No matter how disciplined they are, how well
they plan, or how noble their intentions, dieters will inevitably slip from
time to time. Failure is an inescapable part of the process, and recovering from failure and reasserting discipline is essential for long-term
success. An undertaking as gargantuan as dieting requires a constant
effort over time, and staying true to a dream over the long haul is a key
factor to taking the many small steps leading to the greater goal. While
persistence is a difficult statistic to measure scientifically, I would wager
that the level and longevity of the desire to lose weight in an NWCR
respondent exceeds that of the average obese person. The fact that half
of all people in NWCR report that they're still trying to lose weight
supports this theory.

Clearly, there are general traits and tactics conserved in successful
dieters. However, as evidenced by the ever-expanding waistlines of
Americans, finding a solution to weight problems is less about specific
methodology and more about personalized remedies; no one approach
can work for all people. On this point, I felt that my work was unique:
whereas the standard of the fitness and dietetics communities seemed
to be telling the average dieter *what* to do, I was investigating *how* it
should be done. The following pages contain some of my observations
from the trenches.

## On a Proper Diet

Before I say anything else, it's important to clarify a concept that can have a fuzzy interpretation: what it *really* means to go on a diet. The term has become something of a misnomer. To most people, "going on a diet" conjures visions of a draconian, albeit temporary, state of self-deprivation, where cutting back on the daily quota of treats is rewarded by a steady loss of ounces and pounds. In a stereotypical sense, this is accurate. But what happens after you've lost the weight? Certainly, controlling what and how much you eat is a lifelong process, rather than a temporary affair with defined start and end points. Indeed, the conceptualization of dieting as a transient inconvenience leads to significant difficulties in the formation of a proper attitude for long-term weight management. A more mature understanding of dieting views the process as the beginning of a permanent alteration to one of the most basic components of your lifestyle. To make this even clearer, if you make changes for a while, you may get results, but only for a while. To get long-lasting results, you must make accordingly long-term changes. Viewing a change to your eating habits from a longitudinal perspective can make the decision to diet even more intimidating. It's important not to make the process overly daunting. Diets take time to mature; it's unlikely that you'll immediately adopt the eating habits you will practice ten years down the road. In this light, dieting becomes a series of stepwise alterations, with each change aimed at producing a slightly healthier, leaner person.

The prominent role of diet in daily life makes changing it one of the most challenging lifestyle alterations a person can make. Overeating and eating badly are medically recognized as legitimate disorders. These encompass addiction to and/or dependence on food for a sense of well-being. Thus, when embarking on a diet, you are essentially launching a similar campaign to that of an alcoholic who decides to put down the bottle for good. While struggles to break free of alcohol and drug addiction are well documented, the challenges of combating (over)eating habits are generally not given due consideration. However, one can easily argue that some obstacles associated with dieting equal or exceed those related to battling alcohol and drug abuse.

The major difference between breaking an addiction to a particular substance and embarking on a diet is that it is clinically impossible to quit eating food. To illustrate this point, let us compare hypothetically a smoker who has decided to quit and an obese person planning to lose weight. Practically speaking, the smoker needs to reduce and eventually eliminate his cigarette consumption to achieve his goal. The obese person must continue to eat, but eat less and/or different food in order to become thinner. *He cannot simply abstain from the substances he struggles with; he must learn how to deal with them differently.* In practice, it is a simpler matter for the smoker to remove tempting substances from his life than it is for the dieter to avoid the multitude of widely available junk foods. While other deleterious behaviors can be straightforwardly corrected by quitting, the dieter must not only excise his bad habits but also must replace them with good ones. To do this, a dieter must effect a significant psychological overhaul of his relationship with food. This fact is increasingly recognized by scientists, if not by the commercial diet community. Indeed, recent studies have found improved efficacy in weight-loss programs supplemented with behavior modification therapy.[17] Viewed in this light, dieting becomes inherently more complicated than the comparatively simple act of breaking a particular pattern of behavior, even a deeply ingrained one.

The psychological challenges faced by dieters can be illustrated again by comparing our imaginary smoker and dieter. The smoker's goal is to stop smoking; the dieter's goal is to lose fifty pounds. In their first acts toward their goals, the smoker goes "cold turkey," and the dieter has a bowl of steamed vegetables and goes for a walk. The next morning, both are craving their vices: a pack of Marlboros for the former and a heaping plate of bacon and eggs for the latter. Aside from sheer willpower (an often finite resource), what does each person have in his arsenal to help him battle his cravings? One of the most important psychological tools for lifestyle changes is the ability to validate our actions by examining the results they produce. This common tactic for behavioral reinforcement clearly is more effective in the case of substance addiction. The smoker can now legitimately say, "At this moment, I have accomplished what I set out to do. I am a non-smoker. I have only been one for a day now, and it's still unpleasant, but I have achieved my goal." What can the dieter say to justify his methods? He is still on his diet, and is no doubt suffering as much as the smoker, but he is still fat. He cannot say that he has accomplished his goal or even made significant progress toward it. Thus, a dieter faces the added challenge of staying motivated. As is evident in my account, much of a new dieter's time is spent trying to do just that.

The bottom line here is that a diet has the potential to be one of the hardest things you can ever attempt. Only from understanding and accepting this can the prospective dieter fully appreciate the situation, acknowledging the scope and difficulty of the challenges he faces, and commit to fixing the problem. Succeeding must be your top priority, and must take precedence over other confounding life factors. Though it may sound overly dramatic, when the dieter begins to equivocate, he begins to fail.

## What to Eat

The subject of what constitutes a proper diet is almost immeasurably complicated. Much has already been written about what we should put in our bodies, and not all of it is in agreement. In addition to quantity, the makeup of food is also a complicated subject. Ratios of protein to fat to carbohydrates, processing, the glycemic index, and a million other things have been discussed *ad nauseam*. The result? We know more about food now than ever before, but if you were to poll ten nutrition-ists as to what exactly constitutes a "proper diet," I'd wager you'd get ten different answers.

With so many different opinions, how is it possible to find what is ideal for you? An initial and important consideration is to keep your diet plan (referring here as to what goes in your mouth) as straightforward as possible, without making it overly simplistic. It's easy to get bogged down in the kinetics of metabolism and the biochemistry of nutrition to the point where you can't see the forest for the trees. Often, more is lost than gained with only a partial understanding of the relationships between food, energy, and your body. The layperson usually becomes hopelessly confused, frustrated, or focused on matters of trivial impor-tance. Avoid this by avoiding needless complexity. As someone who's eaten across the spectrum of food options, I've developed my own simple concept of what constitutes proper eating: a good diet is one in which a healthy weight is achieved (or maintained) with a minimum of stress on the body. Note this last bit differs from the mainstream view. Conventional diets seemed aimed at deliberately shocking the dieter by promoting radical changes in eating habits, often in conjunction with the start of an exercise regime. In my opinion, this places far too much stress on average dieters, ultimately leading them to abandon their ef-forts. How healthy is a diet if you can't follow it?

So how do you go about eating to lose weight? In short, you need to gradually implement changes that aren't overwhelming and that you can stick with. Because what acts as a stressor varies from person to per-son, there is no one solution for everyone; it's up to you to find out what works. This means experimentation, which can entail doing odd things or making small changes (which you will later add to as they become ingrained). Even using a drastic diet (e.g., fasting every other day) is acceptable, so long as you intend to modify it to something more man-ageable once you become healthier. I think other authors have covered most of the conventional diet plans, so I instead provide several sample plans that are a little more creative:

### Plan A: The Contingency Plan

Forget about all the other aspects of eating properly EXCEPT hitting your recommended daily intake of unprocessed fruit and vegetables (about nine servings). Eat these first, then eat whatever you want—if you have any room left over, that is. Since consumption of junk food is contingent upon the prior consumption of bulky healthier foods, you may find that you're simply too full to eat the "bad stuff."

### Plan B: The Penalty Plan

Eat whatever you want, but set a weight-loss goal of two pounds a week (or any reasonable number). If you hit your weight, congratulations. If not, fine yourself an amount of money, enough so that you feel the sting. Donate the money to something you really don't care about and wouldn't be inclined to give to otherwise. It seems logical to enlist help with weigh-in/money disbursement duties for this plan, to keep yourself honest. You might be surprised by how far you'll go to protect your money.

### Plan C: The Seth Roberts Approach

Seth Roberts is a psychologist at the University of California, Berkley, who shares my penchant for self-experimentation.[18] One of his experiments dealt with ways to control weight and hunger. Among other findings, Roberts discovered that he could control his cravings for food by ingesting flavorless calories, often something as simple as olive oil. These observations form the basis for his book *The Shangri-La Diet*, a highly controversial work in the nutritional community.

I've never tried any of these diets, and I have no idea if they work. I provide them merely to whet your appetite for creativity. An unorthodox solution may not be necessary for many individuals, but, given the number of people who fare poorly on conventional diets, they might be worth a shot. I'm not advocating a particular plan or path to health or weight loss; I am advocating that you determine for yourself a paradigm that works for you.

This is not to say that there aren't general rules to follow, but there are probably fewer than you think. In the course of my journey, I've discovered a few consistent truths about eating properly that are worth sharing.

First, diet is something that must be actively thought about, especially when you're implementing new changes. There is no way to put this aspect of life on autopilot. And, sad to say, there is no single "perfect" food for everyone, meaning that the selection of a variety of foods is essential and a constant demand. On a larger scale, I have found that dietary requirements change periodically, be it with the seasons, as your body ages, or as your body composition changes. For this reason, I have chosen not to include detailed meal plans of what worked for me. During weight loss, you must also constantly listen to what your body tells you, and examine the trustworthiness of its reports. A *healthy* body knows what it needs, but an overweight body (especially one recently exposed to a new diet) will lie, telling you you're starving when you're not. In the early going, the scale is generally a reliable indicator of whether you're actually going to die if you don't get lunch soon.

Second, continuing in the spirit of variety, everyone differs physiologically, especially with respect to metabolism. We've all seen light eaters who are heavy and enthusiastic devourers of buffets who remain thin. This reinforces the point that *you* must find out for yourself what works for *you*. It's not necessarily easy, and bad decisions are inevitable along the way, but you will build a trustworthy base of knowledge about how to manage your body. This builds on the previous point of listening to your body, as any one person's caloric and nutritive needs tend to be dynamic. When I first began dieting, I had to eat less than normal in order to achieve weight loss. Training for my first triathlon, however, was an intensely demanding experience. I was hungry all the time and would eat far more food than when I was at my heaviest weight. After I adapted to this new workload, my caloric needs subsequently decreased, and I ate less as a result.

Third, eating healthy food is usually more expensive. The abundance of modern food-processing techniques makes preserved foods an inexpensive option. Such items are often tasty but are generally poor fuel for your body. Eating is not a realm unto itself, and financially motivated food selections can have positive or negative implications on other areas of your life. As I became healthier and more active, I had a much harder time handling highly processed foods and would often get an upset stomach if I tried to do too much physical activity after eating them. Bad fuel, bad workout, and the opposite is true as well. Thus, in graduate school, almost a quarter of my budget was spent on purchasing quality stuff to eat. If you're tempted to say, "Yeah, I'll do it later when I can afford it," consider that there are very few things in life that are as permanent as your body. Shouldn't you make it a priority to care for something so fundamental, even if it costs you a few more dollars each day?

Fourth, there are some simple (and painless) changes you can make to your consumptive habits that will help you lose weight. One of the biggest things you can do is to manipulate the amount of energy your body uses to digest food; on average, this energy accounts for about 10 percent of the calories you eat. Each time you eat, your entire digestive system is automatically kicked into action. The more times a day you stimulate this system, the longer it remains active, and the more calories you burn. Eating a meal you normally don't eat (typically, breakfast) and/or eating multiple smaller meals promotes a state of perpetual activity for your digestive machinery. This means that you will burn more energy than you would otherwise, *even if you eat the same number of calories*. Conversely, eating all your calories in one big meal only activates this machinery once, reducing the overall number of calories you burn. In high school, I went through a phase where I ate a single huge meal each day. Even though I was eating less overall, my weight failed to drop, a result that seemed impossible to me. This conservation of weight was at least partly due to my depressed metabolism.

Fifth, and finally, exercise has a massive compensatory effect on what you can get away with eating. This is not always a good thing. Witness my exceptionally poor diet at the start of graduate school, when regular exercise masked my poor eating habits, ultimately holding me back from losing weight. A sedentary person has far less freedom to overeat than an active person. One of the adaptations your body makes as a result of regular exercise is the ability to adjust the rate at which your body burns energy. This allows your body to ratchet up your internal thermostat in response to overeating, burning off the excess calories. Thus, the exerciser receives benefits from regular activity, even when he's not at the gym.

Be realistic: the initial phase of any diet is an acute, drastic process, but in order for your gains to last, this initial period must be followed by a permanent alteration in how and what you eat. My goal was to pursue a high level of fitness (not an aim that I imagine everyone shares), so my diet was shaped to accommodate my athletic endeavors. The typical person undergoes a similar process, albeit on a different scale. While exercise and diet habits are inextricably linked, in a successful lifestyle change, if exercise habits are formed early, the diet will usually fall into place later. It's important to be patient with your diet, as the patterns of what and when you eat take some time to change. What you eat will affect you for the rest of your life, and the time required to modify eating behaviors is worth it in the long run.

For those of you that do seek a similarly high level of fitness (i.e., for competition), diet will come to play an increasingly prominent role in maximizing your athletic abilities. You can get away with eating unhealthy foods and still be reasonably fit, but to reach your full potential you have to be prepared to make some sacrifices in the name of proper nutrition. Strong patterns emerge in dietary requirements for peak fitness, many of which make eating more about fueling and less about taste. Beyond these guidelines, things are again somewhat individualistic. I suggest that the aspiring athlete pay attention to what works and what doesn't with respect to nutrition, particularly before training and races. If you get serious enough, you might want to consider keeping a food journal, using it to correlate what you eat to how you feel during races and key workouts. Using this method, I managed to generate a list of nutritious, clean-burning foods that I could eat with few deleterious effects on my digestive system.

## Exercise

*Things which matter most must never be at*
*the mercy of things which matter least.*

—GOETHE

Without exercise, even the most diligent diet is compromised. I firmly believe that exercise should be immediately introduced into a diet for a complete lifestyle change to occur. You don't need to be in great shape to exercise effectively; running a mile and walking a mile burn about the same number of calories. One just takes longer; the benefits of both can be immediately felt. If you don't think you have the time, just consider the quality and quantity of lifespan you'll potentially add by taking time from other activities to work out regularly.

Exercise should have an equivalent, if not more important, status relative to nutrition in the mind of the dieter. Practically, this means that you need to do some exercise every day (or at least five days a week—that's certainly reasonable). You also need to schedule your exercise wisely; you have to be willing to shuffle other activities around in order to be ready to go when it's time for your workout. If you're a morning person, get up a little earlier to do it then. If you prefer to work out later, make sure you have free time in that part of the day. Don't sabotage yourself by eating heavy, greasy foods that will still be digesting when it's time to work out. Above all, do your scheduled workouts. No skipping. Once you start to slide, it's exponentially more difficult to get back on track than it is to simply stick with a routine.

Exercise is honest; it tells you your fitness level, and quickly. When you get started, there's no such thing as an easy workout or an easy pace. It always feels like your lungs are being seared or your legs are about to fall off. As is the case with controlling your food intake, persistence is key. One day you'll look at your watch, and even though you're still hurting, you'll find that you're going faster or farther or harder than before. Before long, you'll find that workouts geared to your old fitness level are almost comically easy. During training, I would occasionally assume an old running pace just to appreciate how far I had come. Exercise offers frequent positive feedback and motivation. Especially in the early stages, the improvements you make can be rapid and (often) more quantifiable than the effects of dieting.

The bad news is certainly no secret: when you get started, exercising is going to hurt a little. Possibly a lot. It's painful because you have no aerobic capacity to exert yourself, and you're not used to the demands being placed on your muscles and joints. And now the good news: your body will do a hundred little things to help you adapt so that you can stay in motion longer the next time you go out. In addition to metabolizing stored fat calories for energy, your body will build additional blood vessels and increase the amount of oxygen it can process at any given moment. Your muscles will become stronger and more efficient. But even though meaningful changes will occur, they won't all happen overnight, and it's still not going to feel great in the early going. When I first started to exercise, I was sure that there was no way I was going to be able to exercise for long stretches—it was just way too painful. I was perpetually hypoxic, my knees hurt, and I was always really sore when I got up the next morning. But I managed to survive it. You have to trust me—it gets a lot better.

There are also changes that take place above the neck when you exercise. Jerry Seinfeld has a comedy routine in which he questions the point of exercise. As he puts it, the reason to work out is to be in shape … for your next workout. Put in that context, exercising does sound silly, but the question does bear asking: why do such painful things to your body? I think the best answer lies not in the challenge itself but in how you respond to it. When you adopt, take on, and overcome challenges, you're strengthening more than your body. You're developing positive, intangible qualities like tenacity, self-motivation, and, of course, persistence. It doesn't matter if you don't need or want the body of an elite athlete; merely pursuing physical challenges bestows the type of traits that will help you through life and help you feel good about yourself. If you pay attention, you'll usually see that the people who ask what the point of exercising is are those who don't regularly do it.

There are other, less obvious benefits to be gained from exercise. With regard to aging, old people who keep themselves fit are likely to live longer even than those who are a normal weight but don't exercise. When I was a student, I considered pursuing an M.D. and spent a good amount of time in the hospital, where I regularly observed the sick and dying. One thing I learned from my time there was that people rarely drop dead suddenly. More frequently, they develop one or two problems that confine them to a bed and then develop additional comorbidities. People are like horses in this respect: without activity, they tend to physically wilt. Despite this, many people seem to believe that they should take it easier as they get older, as though they need to become less active to live longer. My father, who has counseled individuals in nursing homes, has a favorite piece of advice for living a long, functional life: "Don't lose your legs." If you are still capable of walking, you are probably healthier than someone who isn't. By the same reasoning, if you can run, you're probably better off than a person who can only walk. Rather than resting as you age, you should remain as active as possible for as long as possible. You can outrun death a lot longer if you're in shape.

But what should you do for exercise? If you're seriously overweight and getting started with an exercise program, my advice is simple: just do something. Anything. Walk, run, dance, swim; just get your heart rate up. Your cardiovascular system doesn't know or care what you're up to. All it knows is that it needs to work harder. I particularly recommend the bike for saving your knees and feet. Avid cyclists tend to be very slender, although the bike seat will kill your butt at first. For someone who's looking for efficiency, the best cheap, sustainable, effective activity I know is running. As an ancillary point, I'm not sure I'd recommend starting with running. It can be hard on the unprepared body. For the first few weeks of my running career, I had severe knee pains that magically went away after I lost a little more weight. Finally, as you become more conditioned to the demands of exercise, make it sustainable. Join a sports team, or work to find activities that you like and will continue to do long term. Bottom line: find a way to do something active, and do it every day. For a dieter, as far as exercise is concerned, more is more.

Exercise is a very prominent and very positive manifestation of how a physical change can remake your mental outlook. To be completely honest, when I began exercising, almost every part of me wanted to quit. After a while I got used to it. Gradually, exercise became a neutral activity that simply needed to be done, like taking out the trash. One day, after I'd moved to Florida, thunderstorms prevented me from getting in my daily run. Late that afternoon, I became aware that I was standing at the window, looking wistfully outside like a cat watching a robin at the bird feeder. I had officially come full circle: *not exercising* was now every bit as unpleasant as exercising had been initially. That's where I am still. Sometimes I'll take a day off if I'm tired or banged up, but otherwise, I spend at least a part of every day outside doing some sort of workout.

For those seeking a high level of athletic ability, it's important to remember that what you have driving you is more important than what you have to work with. Along the course of my fitness experiment, I had myself tested for several measures of natural physiological capacities for exercise. Invariably, the test results gave no indication that I was anything but average in almost every way. My ability to absorb oxygen is average, as is my threshold for producing muscle-killing lactic acid. My maximum heart rate is actually below average. The advantages I did have were things that anyone who applies himself can obtain: solid preparation, a lack of ego, and a desire to find a way to do well. As with motivating yourself to stick to a diet, creativity can be essential in inspiring yourself for a workout. Often times in workouts I would rely on positive imagery or use daily sources of stress as fuel. By using these tools in my athletic development, I was able to maximize my performance, even while "trapped" in my unremarkable body.

## Physical Changes

Going from being overweight to a normal weight was a dramatic and wonderful process. At my maximum, I weighed 341 pounds. At my minimum, I weighed 179. That's a loss of 162 pounds, almost half my total bodyweight. As I became a triathlete, I gained some weight back, but I still consider myself more fit than when my weight was lower.

How is this possible? To address this issue, let's discuss the longitudinal changes in my body as I made the transition from big to small and then to truly fit.

Early in a diet, it's OK to be a scale watcher, especially if you're really obese, as I was. The big number on the scale needs to come down. It doesn't matter if the weight you lose is water weight, fat, muscle, internal organs, whatever. Just lose weight. Conditioned by millions of years of evolutionary forces promoting economy, your body, quite against your will, will cling to every last ounce of fat, working to save this precious high-energy substance for a time of true scarcity that will likely never arrive. This being the case, your body will break down any available energy source before it uses fat as a fuel. This includes extra muscle tissue. You'll still to be able to stand up in the morning, but a definite loss of strength often accompanies the early days of a diet. As time passes, your body eventually begins to metabolize fat, and your lost strength returns.

Trainers often recommend a weight-training program for dieters. The idea behind this is that (a) additional muscle helps to burn fat, and (b) added muscle will replace the natural loss of muscle tissue during weight loss. I agree with these assertions to a point: there's nothing wrong with being toned, but building a ton of muscle under a ton of fat seems like nothing more than a recipe to keep strain on your heart and lungs. To a degree, weight is weight. All soft tissue, regardless of the type, requires blood vessels and oxygenated blood, demanding effort from your cardiopulmonary system. When strength training, I use relatively low weights with high repetition counts in order to tone my muscles rather than make them hypertrophic. In this case, less is more.

Shifting from running-only workouts to triathlon resulted in a second change in my body composition. Multisport endurance athletes tend to develop very dense bodies. When I was twelve, I took a swim test as part of a scuba training certification. Part of the test was twenty minutes of treading water. I was delighted to find that my corpulent body floated like a cork. These days, without a full breath of air, I sink to the bottom of the pool like a rock. If you're working out hard and taking care of yourself, an increase in weight does not necessarily mean that you're gaining fat. You may be gaining muscle mass—initially, the same muscle mass you lost in the early part of the diet. Still not reassured? Try measuring your fitness using something other than a scale. Almost any type of physical activity can be quantified (for example, how fast you can run three miles or how far can you swim in ten minutes). When you first begin exercising, pick a test, warm up, and run it to determine your baseline level of fitness. Periodically, run the same test to measure whether you're getting fitter. All else being equal, who's in better shape: the guy who runs three miles in thirty minutes and weighs 150 pounds, or the guy who weighs 155 and runs the distance three minutes faster?

It's not always about how you look in a bathing suit, but you'll probably look good at the pool anyway. All told, I reduced my waist by fifteen inches and switched from XXX-large shirts to mediums (and the occasional small). What was under the hood was also changing. My resting pulse went from seventy beats per minute to a lizard-like thirty-two. My blood pressure, previously borderline high, also changed to reflect my new fitness. My systolic pressure (the first number, the maximum blood pressure that occurs when your heart pumps) actually increased slightly, while my diastolic (or resting) blood pressure was 20 mm Hg lower, suggesting that my heart was really in shape and ready to move oxygenated blood through me at a moment's notice. My cholesterol, previously around 210, dropped to the low 120s, and my triglyceride levels showed similar decreases. My ability to hold my breath (something I frequently measured when bored in class) more than doubled, from sixty seconds to over two-and-a-half minutes. Many people take these "normal" readings for granted, but I can tell you that I appreciate each and every day that I spend free of health problems.

## Mental Changes

Your thoughts and emotions are the essence of your self-perception and outlook on life. Both are influenced by your physical well-being; how you feel about your body significantly affects how you feel about yourself. The rational part of the brain is both stable and positively affected by weight loss. While dieting, if you stick to an effective regimen, monitor your progress, and draw satisfaction from working toward the very logical goal of improving your body's condition, feedback demonstrating your progress should be enough to positively reinforce salubrious behaviors. Emotionally, losing weight can be a surprisingly difficult experience, as you ride an unpredictable rollercoaster of feelings, ranging from pride to frustration to anger to satisfaction. Since the rational and emotional responses of the brain can be diametrically opposed, the feedback you receive from weight loss can be very confusing and often very draining.

A key to success in the mental aspect of losing weight is a willingness to step out of your comfort zones. Comfort zones are not necessarily bad things, but they (by definition) tend to rigidly limit certain aspects of our lives. This can be quite counterproductive if you're in a poor situation to begin with. Weight loss will entail pushing these zones, as will accomplishing almost anything of significance. Use of logic can be of great use in breaking through emotionally defined comfort zones that might otherwise constrain the dieter. Asking yourself (a) what you have to gain or lose from making a change and (b) what you're afraid might happen, is a great way to separate emotional issues from practical ones. As a naturally logical person, I was blessed with the ability to take a hard look at myself and take the next step according to what I saw. There's no denying this was a great advantage in battling a weight problem.

Fear of failure or of making a mistake is often a major barrier to progress. Again, logic is a powerful ally in overcoming this obstacle. Ask yourself, would you be happier trying to make your life better (with the possibility of failure), or living with the feeling that you may be on the wrong path? In conducting my experiment, I failed many times and did many things wrong. While I have mild regrets over the failures, I still think that I proceeded more or less in the best possible manner. It was easy to forgive my foibles because trying and messing up was, in my opinion, far superior to making no effort in the first place. And while I found that it was hard to break out of my comfort zones initially, doing so became far easier once the initial change was made. Once I began losing weight, what was "normal" was now in a constant state of flux. Breaking old habits was like sliding a refrigerator across a floor: hard to get started, but once I got it in motion, pretty easy.

Speaking in the long-term sense, losing weight inspires fantastic feelings. Most of the benefits are obvious: Your confidence increases, especially with members of the opposite sex. You feel better about how you look naked. People do treat you differently. One of the most interesting things that changed as I lost weight was my feelings toward other fat people. Before, I was "one of them" and, as such, usually more than amenable to turning a blind eye to the lifestyle associated with being fat. As I got in better shape, I found it progressively more unsettling that there were people out there who didn't realize just how self-destructive their behaviors could be. And most of all, I became almost overwhelmed by the indifference to well-being I saw in so many people who were literally living dangerously. This indifference is evident in fat and thin people alike, but this situation may soon change. Our society has yet to "officially" stigmatize poor eating and exercise habits as it has done with smoking, but the public consciousness of the consequences of being fat has risen in recent years. Few would argue that large people are not discriminated against in contemporary society. It seems likely that the treatment of obesity will come to follow the trajectory of public attitudes about smoking—a mid-century peak in tobacco use was followed by the castigation of users, following widespread revelations

about the effects of smoking on health. Now smokers are actively perse-
cuted via smoking ban legislation, taxing of cigarettes, and public pressure. Right or wrong, it appears likely that a similar fate may be in store
for obese individuals.

It's important to be honest about the cause of weight gain and obesity. Aside from a handful of rare diseases, there's little reason to become
overweight other than basic self-neglect, usually combined with a dose
of self-delusion. However, there is a decided lack of open societal dialogue on obesity with which self-delusional dieters can remain ground-
ed. I've been on both sides of the coin, and I can tell you that, fat or thin,
you're not doing your huge friend any favors by dancing around the fact
that they are so physically out of whack. I haven't yet met someone who
was truly "fat and happy."

On this last note, I have mentioned several times that heavy people
are often not the best judges of what is going on with their body. This
makes sense: often people who are removed from a situation are capable of seeing it more objectively. Since impartial observers are everywhere, this prompts the question of why fat people often seem unaware
of their plight. At the core of this phenomenon seems to be the thought
process that emerges in the obese. As I encountered overweight people
during my own journey, I noticed that each of them was in some form
of denial, which manifested itself in strange ways. Later, while reading
about the patterns of denial among substance abusers (alcoholics and
drug addicts) I realized that the obese (my former self included) share
this basic mindset.

There are multiple manifestations of denial described in various psy-
chology textbooks. One of the oddest (and possibly most dangerous)
is the concept of fat pride. Organizations with names like the National
Association to Advance Fat Acceptance continue to amaze me.[19] While
it's possible to understand (and even sympathize with) the mentality of
strength in numbers, it is difficult to imagine or comprehend a popula-

tion of people who prefer to define themselves by size alone while promoting an unhealthy body image. But even with such organized groups advocating grossly deviant concepts of fitness, the most pernicious barrier to weight loss remains equivocation on the part of the individual. On the occasions I've ventured outside the bounds of social convention to ask a person about his weight, I've often heard an admission of guilt, even acceptance. This mea culpa is usually attached to a corollary: "Sure I'm fat, BUT…" An excuse in some form inevitably follows. Such people are like slippery politicians—all talk and no action—constantly eluding the reality that they need to make a change. Indeed, talking rather than doing is in many ways worse than doing nothing and keeping your mouth shut.

# The Diet Establishment

*Always listen to the experts. They'll tell you
what can't be done and why. Then do it.*

—ROBERT HEINLEIN

Before deciding to document my own experiences, I first had to wrestle with the question of whether I had anything substantive to add to the mountain of information already out there. After all, I'm by no means an expert, just an average guy who lost a bunch of weight and had a few thoughts after doing so. Has everything worth saying already been said? After poring through a great deal of literature, I have become convinced that very little that has been written about weight loss is useful (or even applicable) to the audience it is intended for. I wondered why so much bad information was out there.

And then I looked at the numbers.

Sixty-five percent of Americans are overweight or obese, with worldwide rates in hot pursuit.[20] In 2003, $93 billion was spent on health care costs directly associated with obesity, with half of that money paid out of programs funded by public tax dollars.[21] U.S. consumers alone spent $55 billion on weight-loss products in 2006.[22] Obviously, the fact that so many of us are big means big business, and many so-called experts have emerged on the topic of being fat and how to avoid it. Usually, these sages fall into two groups. The first subset, usually disguised as objective journalists, focus on selling the gloom-and-doom message of the obesity epidemic and how it's destroying the fabric of our society. This approach is not unlike describing the water to a drowning man: factual, to be certain, but not entirely useful. A preponderance of Americans are aware of the problem, yet the majority of us continue to grow in size. The second group comprises diet gurus and weight-loss specialists. While sharing the enthusiasm of reporters for describing the problem, these experts take the next step by promoting a remedy. Frequently, this happens to be the latest fad diet book or system in which they have a vested commercial interest.

It is an undeniable fact that there are significant economic aspects to all forms of media surrounding obesity and the diet industry. There's an army of people who've built their livelihoods around convincing us that the solution is to listen to them. To protect ourselves, we consumers must examine their agendas. Diet-plan promoters may be well intentioned, but, in providing a commercialized, one-size-fits-all solution, they frequently offer a product that is relevant to many but well suited to none. When I was an undergraduate, a professor of mine explained this phenomenon very well in describing the dilemma of making a commercial dessert that appeals to everyone (I paraphrase): "Say you're in charge of running a company that makes sugary treats. You have only enough machines to produce one dessert, so it must appeal to as broad an audience as possible. Thus, to sell a maximum amount of your product, you design your dessert to include no ingredients that would turn off a segment of the market. You do this at the expense of creating something some people would really love to eat. For example, some folks don't like cinnamon, so you don't put any cinnamon in; others don't like jam, so you don't use jam. In the end, what do you wind up selling? I'll tell you: you get a Twinkie. It's sweet, not too repulsive, and definitely a dessert of sorts, but you would be hard-pressed to find anyone who would proclaim it their all-time favorite."

Using essentially the same approach, diet industry companies have sprung up on the strength of books, plans, programs, or prepackaged food lines, each based around a single "ideal" diet. It's a big pie, and everyone wants a piece. To give you a sense of scope, the U.S. diet industry has projected revenues of $60 billion in 2008, substantially more than will be spent on public research for all other diseases combined.[23] Even though that's a staggering amount of money, it might be worth it if we were getting results in return. But are we? In 2003, Weight Watchers helped fund a clinical study on the benefits of a structured commercial diet plan (including food planning, activity setting, and weekly support meetings) over a self-guided diet (essentially two twenty-minute nutritional counseling sessions and reference to online resources) for moderately overweight people. After the two-year study was completed, the authors concluded that the Weight Watchers plan was superior to a self-guided diet in helping people keep weight off.[24] Or at least, this was what was reported in the media, and, technically, it is true. The actual results of the study, however, leave something to be desired. After two years on a commercial diet plan, an average weight loss of six pounds was reported, compared to only half a pound for the control group. But put this in perspective: the average person in the study was five-foot-six and 208 pounds. Two years of heavily supported dieting resulted in typical commercial dieters trimming themselves to a svelte 202 pounds, comparable to the loss of weight achieved through a professional enema. In this new comparison, Weight Watchers fares less well: their plan takes two years and costs several thousand dollars, while the competition takes an hour and costs fifty bucks. Speaking of finances, Weight Watchers reported 2007 revenues of approximately $1.5 billion, with a gross profit of $814 million.[25]

One of the few points the mainstream diet establishment and I agree on is that a diet is actually a long-lasting set of changes you make in your life. But is commercial dieting really sustainable, or even practical? Say you found it worthwhile to spend several thousand dollars in fees to lose the five or so pounds the average person lost in the previously mentioned study. Your options, according to the company, are (1) continue to follow their program (and continue paying them a significant chunk of change) each year, or (2) don't pay, with the likely consequence of your modest progress evaporating. Is either option particularly palatable? There's a basic truth underlying weight maintenance: your weight is the answer to a simple problem of addition (calories eaten) and subtraction (calories burned). If the sum is negative, you'll lose weight. If it's positive, you'll gain. How much money you pay to do this is up to you, but it has zero impact on the equation.

The profit motive of the diet industry can be illustrated, often comically, by tracking marketing trends. In scrambling to accommodate the latest fads, the weight-loss industry has shown no qualms about contradicting itself in order to sell products. For example, fat was anathema during the 1990s. Almost universally, companies moved to aggressively promote fat-free foods. We gained weight. Ten years later, in a reversal fit to rival those in George Orwell's *1984*, fat is declared to no longer be the enemy; some forms of it are actually healthy, it seems. Now, carbohydrates are the real foe. The same companies that once pushed fat-free bagels are now selling low-carb wraps with equal fervor. We're still getting bigger. I'm waiting for protein-free omelets.

As far as marketing is concerned, most anything is fair game when you're trying to sell stereos or cereal. Should similar rules apply to diet-pill vendors? Weight is a fraught topic for many, and advertising for weight-loss products often appeals to emotion rather than logic. Several disturbing themes recur among advertisements for the diet industry. All too frequently, promotions for weight-loss products imply that there is value attached to being thin. While there's some truth to this, this message can be translated into a personal judgment that is antagonizing and potentially defeating to the dieter in two ways. By saying "thin is good," one implies that "fat is bad." Ergo, "thin people are good," and "fat people are bad." One of the key prerequisites to successfully improving yourself is to believe that you are actually worth improving. If, as an ad suggests, you are a bad person for being fat, what is the point of helping yourself? Worse yet, the company is effectively claiming that their product (i.e., an unproven diet pill) will take the place of more legitimate methods (i.e., diet and exercise). This is, at best, a dubious claim, and, at worst, an unscrupulous one.

Even after you've paid your money, the diet establishment makes great efforts to enlist your loyalty to their system. Weight-loss systems are described in prose suggesting a proprietary quality, implying that the only chance you have to succeed is to rigorously follow their guidelines. One of the most frequently employed tactics to "legitimize" a particular approach is to make the diet sound extremely technical. As a scientist who can generally grasp technical concepts, I feel very strongly that this is done intentionally only to intimidate the layperson into not questioning the basic premise or efficacy of the approach. In the face of so much hype, remember this: our waistlines continue to expand at an alarming rate, regardless of how technically complex the diet establishment manages to make each new iteration of its pitch.

On the topic of communication, I've noticed an apparent disconnect between the givers and takers of diet advice. Too often, I detect a distinct lack of empathy. Experts dictate what must be done without consideration for the difficulty of the prescribed course of action. Imagine walking into a gym for an initial consultation and being double-teamed by a rail-thin nutritionist and a personal trainer with 7 percent body fat, an Adonis physique, and a piece-of-cake attitude. It is easy to imagine how jaded fitness professionals might easily overload the beginner with a barrage of unrealistic expectations. It's a stretch to believe that someone who has spent ten or more years in a world free from restraint will, overnight, effortlessly begin exercising and eating perfectly balanced meals. Again, it doesn't matter how great a program is on paper if no one can stick to it.

Most weight-loss professionals have limited direct experience with the problem they seek to combat. From an economics perspective, this actually makes sense. Would you buy a diet book from a fat guy or take a chubby health reporter seriously? However, from a pragmatic standpoint, the perpetually thin leading the fat has an element of the ridiculous. It's akin to taking dance classes from someone who's seen a lot of Fred Astaire movies; they can tell you what to do, but are ill equipped to show you how. This doesn't invalidate the advice or opinions of the thin or fit—certainly it isn't necessary to have been fat to learn how to be healthy—but it's important to be aware of who is giving you advice and where their experience might be coming from.

Of all my points of disagreement with the diet industry, it is the difference in our respective take-home messages that most compelled me to write this book. Commercial programs prescribe diet and exercise like a recipe. My experiment revealed that pursuing fitness can be a messy business, and the most reasonable path of action cannot be easily encapsulated in the catchy-sounding phrases of diet gurus. In writing this book, I wanted to empower the individual, rather than a corporation. The main factor in any successful drive for self-improvement is rational self-interest. If *you* believe you are ultimately the one responsible for your success or failure, then chances are you will be. My practical goals are twofold: to communicate that you (the dieter) are in control, and to help you consolidate and effectively employ that power. In contrast, commercial weight-loss plans want to convince you that they have all the authority, and they seek to enhance only their powers of control... over you and your pocketbook.

# The Philosophy of Dieting

*Dreams or illusions, call them what you will, they lift us from the commonplace of life to better things.*

—HENRY WADSWORTH LONGFELLOW

Mohandas Ghandi, the renowned spiritual and political leader of India, is known for many reasons, two of the most famous being his pioneering use of nonviolent protest and his embrace of vegetarianism. The interplay between these two factors, however, is less well known. Ghandi was not a vegetarian from birth—quite the opposite, in fact. In his book *Diet and Diet Reforms*, Ghandi recounts how he experimented with eating meat as a child and came to believe that eating meat would help the Indian people to grow strong enough to drive the British away. Fortunately, Ghandi came to embrace the concepts and lifestyle of vegetarianism, and with them, the more peaceful ideals for which he is known. The degree to which the two factors are related is frequently evident in Ghandi's writings; in his book *The Moral Basis of Vegetarianism*, Ghandi speaks at length about how his vegetarian beliefs played a significant role in shaping his personal and political ideations.

If one of history's most significant figures can be so profoundly affected by what he eats, it certainly follows that there exists some interplay between what we eat and the status of our inner moral barometer.

One of the first battles a dieter must undertake is contextualizing and validating the diet within the existing framework of his or her life. The decision to lose weight is a difficult one, requiring much introspection and self-involvement. Without a doubt, there are times during the process when you must make the difficult decision to put yourself and your weight loss first. The resultant feelings of selfishness can be uncomfortable for many people, causing them to abandon their efforts out of a sense of duty to others. Guilty feelings can often be exacerbated by the fact that overweight people may not have a high sense of self-worth to begin with.

Selflessness can be dangerous to a dieter if used to rationalize quitting something beneficial. Think about how many people use altruistic claims as an excuse for their own failings: the father who says he has no time to exercise because he has to take care of his kids, or the mother who can't eat right because she's always at work, providing for her family. In this context, selflessness is just a cop-out to make people feel better about not improving themselves and is really no different from the lies and half-truths that people employ to avoid acknowledging their weight problems. While defined personal principles and a strong constitution are aids to any dieter, a misplaced sense of duty to others can be just as hazardous to an otherwise motivated dieter.

If selflessness puts a damper on weight loss, then the greatest primer for it is a sense of self-worth. Shortly before I decided to diet, I read Ayn Rand's philosophical masterpiece *Atlas Shrugged*. The novel is essentially an exposition of a philosophical and moral system that has at its core the notion of rational self-interest. It was my first introduction to the concept that it might be OK to do something entirely aimed at benefiting myself without feeling guilty or apologetic. This concept is a requirement for successful dieting. Indeed, having a healthy regard for your own value is a critical prerequisite for initiating any self-improvement. How can you be expected to care for something you don't respect? Moreover, the motivation to make positive changes is exponentially more difficult to muster if it does not come from a desire for self-improvement. Recall the unsuccessful diet attempt of my friend Robert, who was driven to diet and exercise to please his girlfriend. His actions were not of his own volition, and I submit that this is why he failed.

Losing weight should be a happy, positive process in the long term, though it can be depressing to suffer in the present for future well-being. When I was going through the rigmarole of losing weight myself, I discovered a few things that kept me mentally and spiritually refreshed when it got tough. These practices might also aid your efforts, if you find them supportive. The keys to staying positive and happy for me were

1. frequently imagining my ideal self;
2. practicing gratitude toward others; and
3. not worrying about things that upset me.

These practices address mental and emotional states that can help or hinder your efforts to improve yourself. First, by imagining yourself in an ideal state, you establish your own optimum situation, which serves as a clearly defined goal to aspire to. Merely by establishing an ideal, you simultaneously motivate yourself and provide an end point to work toward.

The idea of actively expressing gratitude refers to the dieter reaching out to touch the lives of those around them. Ideally, this includes both less fortunate strangers and those you interact with regularly in daily life. The act of volunteering or performing a random kindness has multiple personal benefits and is one of the best things you can do to make yourself feel better *now*. I would often volunteer (often to work with kids) when I felt at my lowest during my diet. When you reach out to strangers in positions less advantageous than yours, you open yourself to two important realizations. First, you have probably done something for them that they cannot do for themselves. This means that you are valuable to them and therefore have value as a person. Second, working with others often exposes you to tremendous acts of human will to succeed and persevere. Together, these two benefits provide infusions of validation and motivation to dieters who might otherwise be foundering for purpose or direction.

The final key to staying positive, not worrying about things that upset you, may not seem pithy in comparison to the other items on the list, but it can be critically important. Worries have a way of magnifying themselves when constantly scrutinized. At the beginning of this book, I described my circumstances before I began to lose weight, which were pretty good by most measures of personal success. Yet at the same time, I was miserably dissatisfied with my life. I had allowed my problems to overwhelm me, and they had grown to dominate and define my existence. Everyone has some problems, but we can largely determine the extent to which our problems affect us. Think about this last point logically: If you get cancer, you can either get chemotherapy, or you can get stressed out and depressed and get chemotherapy. While neither option is desirable, one is clearly preferable. Worry can also serve as a substitute for activity, when we spend our time worrying about the problem rather than searching for the solution.

These principles for staying positive work well for supporting a dieter's overall state of mind, but they're limited in application to smaller practical matters. We are faced with hundreds or thousands of different decisions during a diet, and we must consistently make good choices to continue moving in the right direction. This daily decision making seems to be an Achilles heel for many dieters. To simplify the task for myself, I frequently employed a highly simplified and personalized form of the classic decision-making philosophy called the categorical imperative. The system, created by Immanuel Kant, was originally designed for the weighty problem of determining what is moral.[26] I adapted it for the more pedestrian matter of making everyday diet decisions, but I kept to the same underlying principles. When a question for decision is presented, the possible choices are determined and subjected to a sort of moral calculus, a quick weighing of possible outcomes. According to the theory, the most desirable outcome (and the path you should select) is the one that results in the most "good" or the least "bad" arising from your decision. What is good and bad is, in this case, defined by your diet and your values. For example, picture the all-too-common dilemma of the temptation to cheat on your diet. First, you calculate the good and bad arising from each course of action. It is undeniable that a piece of cheesecake would taste good in the here and now. That immediate satisfaction would be the good result of choosing to eat the cheesecake. On the other hand, there are several bad outcomes associated with this course of action: guilt, the setback to your long-term weight-loss goals, or a possible dietary backslide. After weighing the good and bad outcomes of your other available choices, you may decide to allow yourself this indulgence, stay fast to your long-term goal, or compromise and only eat half a piece of cheesecake.

As you can see, by applying this system, you must search for and evaluate all the possible solutions to your problem and then think about both the short- and long-term implications of your potential actions. While it only takes a moment, I find this exercise very valuable in enhancing my decision-making skills, a fundamental component in making wise choices in life. In this context, having a clearly defined long-term goal (and how much it means to you in comparison to a quick bite of something tasty) is a superb way to keep your priorities in perspective.

Taken together, the three principles for mental well-being and the decision-making system I have advocated constitute a basic philosophical tool kit for staying positive and making good decisions, with the ultimate goal of losing weight and (hopefully) becoming happier as a result. Why is being happy relevant to dieting? Simply put, a sad, un-motivated person is likely to continue to wallow in self-pity and apathy, while a happy, motivated person is likely to proactively manage their life and develop strategies to succeed and flourish. In this way, good decision-making and personal well-being are integrally related to one another. I learned this the hard way in college as I allowed myself to deteriorate slowly, both physically and mentally, through inaction.

# Social Aspects of
# Weight Loss

*To avoid criticism, do nothing, say nothing,
be nothing.*

—ELBERT HUBBARD

In 1995, the National Academy of Science issued a report summarizing the current methods for preventing and reversing obesity.[27] Included in the report was a list of positive and negative predictors for individual success on various diets. While many of the positive and negative predictors were things that one might expect to see, a surprising negative predictor was repeated attempts to lose weight. To paraphrase the authors of the study, those who failed to lose weight on their initial attempt were statistically less likely to ever lose weight. I wondered why this was. Was a second or third attempt at weight loss harder than the initial one? If I could discover why, I might gain some valuable insight into the act of dieting. People constantly in the throes of weight loss and gain began to fascinate me. I called these people "yo-yo dieters" and began to study why they did what they did.

To me, yo-yo dieters were a curious breed, both capable and decadent in nature. Unlike those who flatly failed to lose weight, these individuals clearly possessed some amount of efficacy and willpower. However, despite these positive traits, this population was clearly lacking in some regard, as they all were prone to regaining all the weight they had worked hard to lose. This made little sense to me. Losing and then regaining weight put them in essentially the same boat as those who stayed rotund consistently. Why would they bother with the unpleasantness of dieting? And wouldn't these individuals eventually learn how to keep weight off once they lost it? In pondering the issue, I arrived at only two rational explanations to account for yo-yo dieting. The first possibility was a procedural problem: yo-yo dieters might subscribe to unsustainable weight-loss tactics. This possibility seemed unlikely to account for every failed diet; I'd seen yo-yo dieters employ an impressive variety of approaches to weight loss, and many were successful in using many different diets (on different occasions) to lose weight. This suggested that the problem was not in their methods, but in their attitudes. A second possibility occurred to me: yo-yo dieters care about losing weight, but aren't concerned with keeping it off.

I began to create a theory, the central premise of which was the notion that yo-yo dieters lost weight solely to earn the praise of others. This is hardly unheard of; to see the lengths to which individuals will go to earn external praise, one need only think of the parent-child relationship. Operating under a desire for external affirmation, yo-yo dieters lose weight, often rapidly and in substantial quantity. Weight loss is, as a rule, rewarded with praise by friends, family, and even strangers. But what then? After the weight disappears, no one is there to constantly tell the yo-yo dieter that they still look good. Without the continual affirmation from others, the impetus is lost and the weight is regained. While we are generally quick to offer praise to someone who has lost weight, no one is likely to criticize the same person's backslide into obesity. Once heavy again, the yo-yo dieter repeats the sequence *ad infinitum*. Though this theory is difficult to prove, thinking about yo-yo dieters was the first time that the influence of social interaction on weight loss truly became apparent to me. Although the undertaking to lose weight will always be an individual one, the process does not occur in the absence of input from others.

Communicating openly about weight problems is difficult. Any discussion of an individual's size—especially in that individual's presence—is a sensitive matter. As I was growing up, few of those around me were willing to tell me flat out that I was enormous. Even good friends were willing to absorb my poor mood and watch me physically deteriorate but unwilling to say anything for fear of appearing boorish or insensitive. Sugarcoating or altering truths about an individual's weight might be socially preferable, but it does nothing to correct the propensity of the overweight to delude themselves. Make no mistake: being overweight IS bad for you. Don't kill the messenger. Obesity negatively affects quality of life (both mentally and physically) more than any other single health problem. Anything we can do to head it off is, in my book, worthwhile.

On a societal level, we Americans often contradict ourselves on the issue of weight control. We send mixed messages, beginning in the formative years. For example, take physical fitness and health education in public schools. While providing physical fitness classes and teaching the rudiments of proper diet are required by every curriculum, schools often subvert their own message with what they serve to eat. Increasing reliance on commercial vendors has flooded schools with incredibly unhealthy lunches and snacks. The result: kids stuffed with pizza and French fries, trudging into PE class. The conflict between curriculum and cafeteria menu sends a confusing message on the value of fitness.[28]

We send similar mixed messages in talking about weight loss. Confronting the problem of weight is difficult, as obesity remains something of a taboo subject in our ultra-sensitive society. Few people seem willing to connect the problem of being overweight and the overweight individual. For example, people frequently discuss studies in the news linking obesity to (pick your disease), but not with their obese friend.

Instead of talking openly and seriously about weight problems, people make immature jokes, which fat people hear and become defensive about. It's unsurprising, then, that when someone has the temerity to talk openly about obesity with a heavy person, the heavy person becomes defensive, bristling at what they perceive as an impending insult or patronizing advice. Until we resolve these communication issues, open dialogue on the obesity epidemic may remain elusive.

Most of the stuff that is said is about weight change is positive, like telling a dieter that he or she "looks great." Still, people have some strange ideas and when you're dieting they can be adept at finding a "polite" way to express their opinions about what you're doing. Amazingly, I've actually heard people actively discouraging motivated dieters. I call these people "doubters." Even if you're good friends with a doubter, it's hard to believe these kinds of people have your best interests in mind. I can't think of any reasons people would seek to derail an otherwise committed individual from a fruitful pursuit. Perhaps they perceive heavier individuals as occupying a lower social position than themselves and seek to maintain this status quo. Perhaps they're heavy themselves and are uncomfortable with your metamorphosis (more on this later). Perhaps they're just ignorant to the dangers and social detriments to living life as an overweight person, and, upon seeing you struggle, think you'd be better off staying "fat and happy."

Doubters usually begin their pitch under the guise of legitimate concern. "Are you sure that's healthy?" they often say as a prelude to voicing their opinion of what you're doing. A doubter can be easily discerned from a curious person making a simple inquiry; the former will not be interested in what you have to say about your diet (their mind is likely already made up), while the latter will be ready to listen. The negativity a doubter projects does no one any good. When confronted by those who would seek to hold you back, it's important to remind yourself that what you're doing has tremendous value, and that any person willing to work against that is essentially not a good influence. If you explain this to them, and they fail to respect your wishes, ask yourself if it's really worth involving them in your life at this time.

Friendships are generally maintained and often strengthened in the face of ongoing weight loss, with one common exception: overweight friends who remain fat as you continue to lose weight. Many times, fat friends suddenly become doubters as you begin to make progress. In my estimation, this is more understandable (if not entirely logical) than when skinny people attempt to block or trivialize your loss of weight. You must remember that you may now scare your larger acquaintances. When you were obese, your presence may have made them feel more secure about the social acceptability of their own body size. Perhaps they think you're trying to be "better" than them by being thinner, or are somehow "betraying" them in some ill-defined manner. Most of all, they may be worried that you will cease to be their friend as you become thinner and will begin treating them as they are frequently treated by society in general. These feelings are driven by simple self-interest, the irrational counterpart to the feelings of self-preservation that probably drove you to lose weight, and not by malicious intent. When confronted by this situation, I suggest treating your larger friend a bit more delicately than a typical doubter. Honest communication is always preferable to estrangement. Pay it forward by explaining what makes you passionate about losing weight and try to recruit your friend to join you. At worst, she'll understand your motives. Why isolate a person when you can empower her and make a closer friend? I actually had several overweight friends tell me I was a role model to them for trying to lose weight. Being told that someone looks up to you is perhaps the greatest single motivation to stay on the straight and narrow path to successful and permanent weight loss.

Support systems also remain critical to successfully effecting a lifestyle change. I was always predisposed toward extreme self-sufficiency in all my undertakings, which might suggest that the majority of strategizing and hard work I did while losing weight was performed in absolute isolation. In practice, nothing could be further from the truth. I relied heavily on a small group of people for a huge variety of needs. Even though no one can run a mile or skip a meal for you, involving others can be a great way to alleviate some of the common difficulties you face when dieting. Besides the obvious benefits of advice, pep talks, positive (and negative) feedback, and solidarity (as in the case of running buddies or sympathy dieters—those who are generous enough to eat by choice what you eat by personal mandate), there are less obvious advantages to relying on others. Merely revealing your weight-loss plan to a family member or good friend brings a measure of accountability to your actions: you must now back up what you've said publicly if you don't wish to appear a failure. Your creativity is the only limit in this regard; more extroverted people might rely on their social networks even more heavily for support. Just remember that you're probably going to be a little cranky during the early phases of your diet, and if you want to continue to have a social network you'd better learn to disappear when you get really ticked off from several weeks of frequent hunger pangs.

While I controlled the number of people whom I voluntarily involved in my effort, there were many others who influenced me in ways I would never have imagined when starting out. Even people who had no direct role in my efforts had an effect. For example, examining the differences between those who succeeded and those who failed at their own diets had a tremendous impact on my own techniques and belief systems. People have an inherent ability to clearly see situations in which they are not involved, and watching strangers was often particularly useful to the scientist in me for crystallizing an abstract process or idea. One day, long after I'd lost weight, I was at the grocery store, in the frozen foods section. I had been toying with the idea of writing about my experiences, and I was stuck struggling to reconcile how reasonably intelligent people become and remain so terribly overweight in light of the detrimental consequences. The possibilities overwhelmed me. Were we all dumber than I thought? Blind to the facts? In a state of active or passive denial? I couldn't come to a solid conclusion by looking at my own life. As I pondered the question, a gentleman in a motorized scooter turned into the opposite end of my aisle. This fellow's girth made my weight problem seem comically miniscule in comparison. As he reached into the grocer's case to add a brace of frozen pizzas to his cart, I saw the slogan emblazoned on the front of his tent-sized T-shirt. In bright green letters, it read proudly: "I Beat Anorexia." Though I saw the humor in this tongue-in-cheek message, a deeper thought struck me. *This shouldn't be funny. This dude's about fifty calories from keeling over and being the story in the paper tomorrow morning that people will laugh over.* Just like that, I had my revelation: this guy had no earthly idea just how badly off he was. With that, I began to think about how individuals turn a blind eye to their physical failings. That night, I began scribbling the first of many notes that became the basis for this book.

## Conclusions

*Until one is committed there is always hesitancy,*
*There is one elementary truth, the ignorance of which kills*
*Which no man could have dreamed would come his way.*
*Whatever you can do or dream you can, begin it.*
*Boldness has genius, power and magic in it.*

—GOETHE

When writing up any scientific investigation, the end is where one lists and discusses the conclusions drawn during the investigation. In many measurable ways, my experiment was a success: I'd gone from the deepest, darkest depths of physical decrepitude to the heights of athletic competition. By changing my body, I'd changed far more than just how big or small I was; I'd improved my mind, my outlook on life, and a hundred other things as well. Certainly, if one person can do it, that bodes well for everyone else. But it's more complicated than that. As is often the case in scientific research, it seems that this investigation has raised at least a few new issues.

One of those questions is what's next. I certainly have room for improvement: even though I won my division at nationals, I was eighty-seventh overall, so there's little chance of my reaching the very top of the mountain anytime soon. Even so, if there's one thing I've learned, it's that you can never say anything for sure. How far can I take what I'm doing? I have no idea, but I'm still committed to finding out. When you don't try, the only thing you gain is a certainty about what's going to happen: absolutely nothing. In that light, uncertainty is positively liberating. I've learned that attempting something, no matter how ambitious, brings into play the possibility that you'll manage to do it. That's what all of this is about, really: chasing possibilities.

I have reached a few solid conclusions. My firsthand experiences have increasingly led me to agree with the notion that obesity is indeed a disease, one that contributes to and ties together many physical, mental, and social problems. It's also a disease many of us will be forced to reckon with. Obesity is shockingly widespread and has increasingly impacted our society and quality of life. A controversial 2005 study in the New England Journal of Medicine suggested that, for the first time in recorded history, the current generation may have a shorter life expectancy than the previous one.[29] Obesity is a unique disease: the remedy is often obvious, cheap and relatively easy to prescribe, yet few succeed in conquering the condition. Rather than the cold facts about weight loss, many of us find ourselves more concerned with the daily personal problems that seem to accompany our expanding waistlines. A weight problem doesn't give you anywhere to hide. It can't be negotiated with, cajoled, or dumped on someone else. It's a personal test in the truest sense.

The cure can be as challenging as the disease is pernicious. Along the way, I learned that weight loss is tougher than I ever imagined. To combat obesity, you need your brains, your passion, and your experiences to guide you. How you respond to the challenge, in my opinion, reflects on your character. It's a big deal. You have to go out and make it happen. Extraordinary results have come from people creating things out of nothing: great literary masterworks, advances in science, technology, and medicine. Even systems of government evolve in such a manner. No great achievement can be accomplished without three things: application of reason, great effort, and failures along the way. Persistence, when combined with a vision and a tolerance for failure, can result in some really amazing things happening, from individual accomplishments to collaborations of the grandest scale.

What of the main question, the hypothesis that I spent so many hours, days, and years testing? Are we a slave to our genes and our history, or can our free will, logic, and determination be enough to overcome our innate proclivities? The answer, I have concluded after careful consideration, is a qualified "yes" to the latter proposition. The traits we humans have come by more recently—our power of choice and our faculty of reason—are strong enough, if applied properly, to overcome our deepest instincts, habits, and rituals. People have often asked me why I would take my experiment so far. After all, most people have no aspirations beyond losing a few pounds and keeping them off. To them I say this: the reason I traveled so far along the spectrum of fitness was not to set a precedent for others to follow, but to demonstrate that it was *possible*. In other words, my goal is not to set a standard, but to discourage arbitrary self-imposed limits.

None of this is to say that someone with more modest goals is on easy street. If you look around, this should be apparent. Our vestigial programming to retain weight is strong, stronger than our reason or de-sire separately. It is only when we combine these two faculties smartly and efficiently that our brains can fool our biology and get us where we want to go. *How* to go about applying our best traits to defeat some of our worst (both biological and less tangible traits like laziness) is the real question. It's a question that I believe has not yet been explored fully. Of course, our best and worse traits play an integral role in defin-ing us as people. Regardless of the features that make us who are, it's what we choose (or don't choose) to do that makes us the people we become.

Always remember that human beings are dynamic entities. We're rarely at a standstill; all of us are either getting better or getting worse, improving ourselves or letting ourselves rot. Whether you move for-ward or backward is, ultimately, up to you. As they say, the ball's in your court.

# NOTES

1. Fritsch J. "95% Regain Lost Weight. Or Do They?" *New York Times,* May 25, 1999.

2. For information about trends on spending toward weight-loss products and/or services, see

Rippe JM. "Overweight and health: communications challenges and opportunities." *Am J Clin Nutr* 1996;63:Suppl:470S-473S.

Kuczmarski RJ, Flegal KM, Campbell SM, Johnson CL. "Increasing prevalence of overweight among US adults: the National Health and Nutrition Examination Surveys, 1960 to 1991." *JAMA* 1994;272:205-211.

"The painful business of losing weight." *The Economist.* August 30, 1997:45-7.

3. Stunkard A, McLaren-Hume M. "The results of treatment for obesity: a review of the literature and report of a series." *AMA Arch Intern Med.* 1959 Jan;103(1):79-85. Though somewhat dated in methods, this study was one of the first and most widely-reported studies on the difficulty in losing weight.

4. National Center for Health Statistics. *Chartbook on Trends in the Health of Americans.* Health, United States, 2006.

5. Hensrud DD, Weinsier RL, Darnell BE, Hunter GR. "A prospective study of weight maintenance in obese subjects reduced to normal body weight without weight-loss training." *Am J Clin Nutr.* 1994 Nov;60(5):688-94.

6. Sui X, LaMonte MJ, Laditka JN, Hardin JW, Chase N, Hooker SP, Blair SN. "Cardiorespiratory Fitness and Adiposity as Mortality Predictors in Older Adults." *JAMA* 2007; 298(21):2507-2516.

7. Those statistics are compiled from the following studies:

Blair SN, Shaten J, Brownell K, Collins G, Lissner L. "Body weight change, all-cause mortality, and cause-specific mortality in the Multiple Risk Factor Intervention Trial." *Ann Intern Med* 1993;119:749-757.

Horm J, Anderson K. "Who in America is trying to lose weight?" *Ann Intern Med* 1993;119:672-676.

Lissner L, Odell PM, D'Agostino RB, et al. "Variability of body weight and health outcomes in the Framingham population." *N Engl J Med* 1991;324:1839-1844.

Thomas PR, ed. *Weighing the options: criteria for evaluating weight-management programs.* Washington, D.C.: National Academy Press, 1995.

Williamson DF, Pamuk E, Thun M, Flanders D, Byers T, Heath C. "Prospective study of intentional weight loss and mortality in never-smoking overweight US white women aged 40-64 years." *Am J Epidemiol* 1995;141:1128-1141.

8. This study was eventually published (Anson RM, Guo Z, de Cabo R, Iyun T, Rios M, Hagepanos A, Ingram DK, Lane MA, Mattson MP. "Intermittent fasting dissociates beneficial effects of dietary restriction on glucose metabolism and neuronal resistance to injury from calorie intake." *Proc Natl Acad Sci U S A.* 2003 May 13;100(10):6216-20). Note that the published study does not match the description on which my subsequent calculations were based, likely because of miscommunication or misunderstanding at the time. However, I later discovered that other studies found differences in body weight on intermittent fasting. E.g., Masoro EJ, Yu BP, Bertrand HA. Action of food restriction in delaying the aging process. Proc Natl Acad Sci U S A. 1982 Jul;79(13):4239-41.

9. A number of studies have found a wide array of of health problems, including premature death, in jumbo-sized football players.

10. "Doctoral Candidate Recipient Characteristics," *Chronicle of Higher Education.* http://chronicle.com/

11. These feelings are similar to those reported by filmmaker Morgan Spurlock during his month-long diet of exclusively fast food, undertaken for his documentary *Super Size Me.*

12. Karlsson J, Taft C, Rydén A, Sjöström L, Sullivan M. "Ten-year trends in health-related quality of life after surgical and conventional treatment for severe obesity: the SOS intervention study." *Int J Obes* (Lond). 2007 Aug;31(8):1248-61.

13. I later learned that shaving your legs does not make you more aerodynamic—it is done to make abrasions incurred while cycling heal more easily.

14. "Doctoral Candidate Recipient Characteristics," *Chronicle of Higher Education*. http://chronicle.com/

15. http://www.nwcr.ws/

16. Klem ML, Wing RR, McGuire MT, Seagle HM, Hill JO. "A descriptive study of individuals successful at long-term maintenance of substantial weight loss." *Am J Clin Nutr* 1997;66:239–46.

17. For example, Wadden TA, Sternberg JA, Letizia KA, Stunkard AJ, Foster GD. "Treatment of obesity by very low calorie diet, behavior therapy, and their combination: a five-year perspective." *Int J Obes*. 1989;13 Suppl 2:39-46.

18. For example, Roberts S. "Self-experimentation as a source of new ideas: ten examples about sleep, mood, health, and weight." *Behav Brain Sci*. 2004 Apr;27(2):227-62

19. An actual organization: http://www.naafa.org/.

20. Ogden CL, Carroll MD, Curtin LR, McDowell MA, Tabak CJ, Flegal KM. "Prevalence of overweight and obesity in the United States, 1999-2004." *JAMA*. 2006;958(13):1549-1555.

21. Finkelstein EA, Fiebelkorn IC, Wang G. "National medical spending attributable to overweight and obesity: how much, and who's paying?" *Health Aff* (Millwood). 2003 Jan-Jun;Suppl Web Exclusives:W3-219-26.

22. *The U.S. Weight Loss & Diet Control Market* (9th Edition). Marketdata Enterprises, Inc.

23. *The U.S. Weight Loss & Diet Control Market* (9th Edition). Marketdata Enterprises, Inc.

2007 and National Institutes of Health: Annual Research Budget. http://www.nih.gov/.

24. Heshka S, Greenway F, Anderson JW, Atkinson RL, Hill JO, Phinney SD, Miller-Kovach K, Xavier Pi-Sunyer F. "Self-help weight loss versus a structured commercial program after 26 weeks: a randomized controlled study." *Am J Med*. 2000;109(4):282-7.

25. United States Securities and Exchange Commission: Financial Statement for Weight Watchers International, Inc., for 12 months ending 12-29-07.

26. Immanuel Kant. *Groundwork of the Metaphysics of Morals*. Cambridge University Press. 1998.

27. National Academy of Sciences piece on obesity treatment. *Weighing the Options: Criteria for Evaluating Weight-Management Programs*. National Academy of Sciences Institute of Medicine, 1995. http://books.nap.edu/catalog/4756.html

28. The evolution of school lunch is discussed in Greg Critser's *Fat Land: How Americans Became the Fattest People in the World* (Houghton Mifflin, 2003)

29. Olshansky SJ, Passaro DJ, Hershow RC, Layden J, Carnes BA, Brody J, Hayflick L, Butler RN, Allison DB, Ludwig DS. "A potential decline in life expectancy in the United States in the 21st century." *N Engl J Med*. 2005 Mar 17;352(11):1138-45.

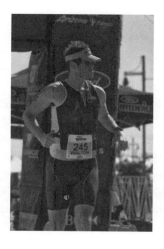

## ABOUT THE AUTHOR

Noah Walton received his undergraduate degree in biology from Duke University and his PhD in neurobiology from the University of Florida. After postdoctoral training at the University of Chicago, Noah is now a scientist in the San Francisco Bay area, where he leads a dual life as an athlete and scholar, competing in triathlons while publishing scientific studies. His scholarly work has been featured on CNN and in *Scientific American* and *The New York Times*.

The legitimacy of the scientific aspects of the Noah's foray into weight loss are underscored by his proven track record in biomedical research, where he has published numerous papers in top-tier scientific journals and presented work at international conferences. He effectively transformed himself from a couch potato to an athlete who qualified for, and succeeded in, the 70+ mile US National Triathlon Championships. He has completed 2 Ironman (140+ miles) races, 6 half-Ironmans, and a several marathons in the past 3 years. He lives in San Jose, California.

Noah's website is www.noahmwalton.com.

Sentient Publications, LLC publishes books on cultural creativity, experimental education, transformative spirituality, holistic health, new science, ecology, and other topics, approached from an integral viewpoint. Our authors are intensely interested in exploring the nature of life from fresh perspectives, addressing life's great questions, and fostering the full expression of the human potential. Sentient Publications' books arise from the spirit of inquiry and the richness of the inherent dialogue between writer and reader.

Our Culture Tools series is designed to give social catalyzers and cultural entrepreneurs the essential information, technology, and inspiration to forge a sustainable, creative, and compassionate world.

We are very interested in hearing from our readers. To direct suggestions or comments to us, or to be added to our mailing list, please contact:

## SENTIENT PUBLICATIONS, LLC

1113 Spruce Street
Boulder, CO 80302
303-443-2188
contact@sentientpublications.com
www.sentientpublications.com